D0065174

To Ann

Happy Reading!

POINTS of
ORIGIN

[signature]

10-26-2006

All of the characters in this book are fictitious, and any resemblance
to actual persons, living or dead, is purely coincidental.

Ponder House Press
2565 Lake Circle
Jackson MS 39211-6625

Layout and Design by The Gibbes Company

ISBN-10: 0-9771126-1-6

ISBN-13: 978-0-9771126-1-6

First Edition

Printed in Canada

To those who give second chances.

Acknowledgments

Those of us from around here know that the South is filled with sincere individuals willing to help with noble causes. Whether or not writing fiction novels qualifies as such may be a matter of opinion. Nevertheless, let's assume *Points of Origin* and its older sibling *House Call* are eligible, making me obliged to more sincere people than I could ever list. But I am going to try.

First of all, much is owed Sally North, my lovely wife of twenty-seven years. Sally's help in completing the eleventh-hour revisions to the manuscript of *Points of Origin* resurrected for me fond memories of simpler times when we worked together on *The 1978 Ole Miss*, our university yearbook. That's when the deal was made. To my son William and daughter Anderson, I give my loving thanks for tolerating a father who is a full-time physician and aspiring author. Likewise, I remain indebted to my mother Evelyn Hays North for her diligent assistance and encouragement. As a writer, it is certainly helpful to have a wife and a mother who are both English teachers.

The completed manuscript of *Points of Origin* was edited separately and painstakingly by Karen Cole, MD; Helen DeFrance; Mona Evans; Nan Graves Goodman; Edra Kimmel, MD; and Tom Shelton, as well as by Sally and Evelyn North, all having an amazing eye for detail and the brains to match.

Several key individuals provided research expertise in completing this book, which is not intended to be an authoritative source on any subject. Among the gifted saints who shared their knowledge with me were Edra Kimmel, MD; Bill Kimmel; Alan Stallings, MD (aviation); Leslie Decareaux, Kirk McDaniel, John Grimes, Ricky Dawson, Missy Welch Ross (fire science); Pippa Jackson (building materials salvage); Scott Runnels, MD (plastic surgery); Cesar Lopez; James Tomek, PhD (foreign languages); Charlie Molpus (golf); and Helen DeFrance, Leslie Carpenter (culinary artistry). Any mistakes regarding those aforementioned topics, as well as any other errors in this novel, belong to me – but I dare you to find any.

Other special thanks is due the employees and fellow physicians of the Jackson Healthcare for Women, PA., as well as those of area hospitals and other medical offices.

The following individuals have also been invaluable in my writing and publishing exploits: Claire Aiken; Carole Bailey; Jim Blackwood; Lieutenant Billy Brown; Marsha Cannon; Sylvia Carraway; Pat and Bruce Crain; Wray Eidt; Rita Farmer; Betty Fortenberry; Jane Gonzalez; Duke Goza, JD; Denise Grones; Darlene Herring; Toni Irby, LPN; Wanda Jewell; Kim Jurgens; Phoebe Kruger; Luke Lampton, MD; Ann Lee; Bill Lowther; Anne Marion; Len Martin; Diana McDiffett; Gayden Metcalfe; Margaret Monger; Joel Payne, MD; Barbara Phillips; Tricia Redditt; George Ritter, JD; Josh Robinson; Ellen Rolfes; Mary Shapley; Dorothy Shawhan; Mary Lou Webb; and Ben Yarbrough, MD.

Furthermore, the many booksellers and libraries who continue to welcome my works onto their shelves and sponsor author appearances are special friends as are the members of the local and region media. I continue to appreciate, as well, the emails, surface notes, and other comments from readers. Please keep them coming.

Also to Darrell Wilson, president of the Repair Team, thank you for your kindness and style. Finally, Denton Gibbes and the creative staff of The Gibbes Company deserve my heartfelt gratitude for this novel's design and the guidance that pushed along its creation.

PROLOGUE

The newspaper obituary was poorly written. Even my tenth grade education picked up the grammatical flaws, not to mention the rambling content and elementary sentence structure: at least two run-ons and way too many commas. Although there was a subject-verb disagreement toward the close of the piece, misspelling was not an issue; I guess the *Larkspur Ledger* mercifully ran it through spell-check. No doubt the bereaved, overwhelmed author could have benefited from such a book as *Obituaries for Idiots* or perhaps a Google search for tips on writing death announcements. Unfortunately, that long column, an eruption of gut-wrenching sadness and bitterness, would be just the first of two the writer would ultimately pen.

Running alongside several others that day in the newspaper, the obituary mentioned the immediate family as survivors as though merely a single group was devastated. By anyone's standards, the lives of at least four families (maybe just two families, depending on how you define *family*) were affected by the death – certainly more than four if one counts the physicians who eventually had to leave town over it. The funny thing about that hastily drafted, redundant memorial was that the paper did not bother to mention those other families, who in a liberal sense were just as immediate as the blood relatives of the deceased. Their existence, too, was twisted, no, tormented by one act, one day, one death.

The two years that followed found me as a high school senior in Larkspur, Mississippi. Normally that period of a teenager's life would be a joyous relief, a climactic ritual to the great American educational experience. But for me, remembrance of that phase still evokes a sadness that has never found resolution. Sometimes the grief reaches a degree that is more than intolerable, depending upon how I remember my parents and how I believe others judge their final circumstances.

Many times the anguish of such regret causes mere existence to become marginal at best, especially when regret becomes a way of life.

And that existence was consumed by more calamity. Sometimes I have referred to those other sordid catastrophes as the *rest of the stuff*: the misfortune of stooped-over Mrs. Architzel and her dog; my police arrest with sexy Kaylee; the bloody mess in that serene neighborhood rose garden; and the other tripped-up actions that led to my wearing the proud uniform – the uniform of the Larkspur City Fire Department.

Nonetheless, during that coveted night spent on the hill with society's upper crust, the distinguished uniform was left hanging in my closet, along with its spare.

Contents

POINTS of
ORIGIN

◆ ◆ ◆

DARDEN NORTH, MD

Chapter
1
•••
THE DESERVING

Anyone in the squirming audience who was forced to listen could have written the annual address.

"I challenge you to a sacrifice that is more than financial, a true spiritual, emotional sacrifice. Many of you have already made the ultimate commitment to the youth of Larkspur and the surrounding community. Through your tuition dollars and tax-deductible donations, your children have received the highest quality high school education available anywhere. After enrolling your sons and daughters at Larkspur Christian Academy, you immersed them in a secondary curriculum that will ultimately prepare them, actually over-prepare them, for any college or university in this country." The headmaster pressed on for the kill. "And all the while during this high school experience, a true sense of integrity and honesty has been molded into our students as they have made their walk with God at Larkspur Christian Academy."

His custom was to pause at this moment for prayer, an intriguing habit for someone who had not seen the inside of a church or touched a Bible in at least twenty years. However, that night Mr. Gregory Whitestone was running short on time and omitted a direct appeal for God's blessing. "In its constant march to provide superior higher education, year after year our faculty has stimulated graduates to reach for diversity, moving toward challenging careers. Those choices have pushed them well beyond the borders of Mississippi.

"For that reason the board of directors has voted to change the name of our facility to Larkspur Institute for Education." There would have been a hush of surprise at the announcement except that the audience members, as well as those of us sitting on stage, were nearly asleep. "This modern moniker will reflect not only the kindness and compassion that composes the moral fiber of our teachers and administrators, but will also clarify our quest to maintain academic excellence."

Gregory Whitestone concluded the commencement address, calling for the audience's greater commitment to God, democracy, family, and intellect – a loyalty automatically endorsed by school support. Whether it was a high school graduation exercise like mine, a football game, an annual honors day program, senior dance recital, or local civic club, Mr. Gregory Whitestone remained steadfast. To the listener he stressed no greater goal for mankind than prayerful, financial support of the newly-renamed private school.

I recall sitting there in the number one chair, hoping that I was listening to Whitestone for the last time and thinking about the financial cost of my senior year: seventy-five hundred dollars plus. While my grandfather would more likely have enjoyed spending that chunk on something else – like an investment or another memorial for my parents – he certainly did not begrudge the expense to educate me at Larkspur Christian – I mean Larkspur Institute for Education. In a happier time during the years before my senior year, when Mom and Dad had no real financial concerns and they paid the tuition, my parents could have spent the money on a getaway vacation or a piece of jewelry.

Those of us stiffly propped on that auditorium stage, in a hall which also doubled as a basketball court, were forced to attention during Whitestone's oration. In addition to being on display in front of a proud, anticipatory crowd, the scratchy graduation gowns were a perpetual stimulant, fortunately enough as to keep each wearer from dozing off and sliding out of his or her chair.

His seat was well below the thin stage, toward the back of the area roped off for the rest of the seniors, the ones whose class rank was significantly lower. Although his gown was just as uncomfortable as those of the honor students, it was garnished only with nondescript tassels. The scarcity of gold tassels like those flowing from the smart kids was not a concern. The nobility, or lack of it, was lost on him.

He thought about the fire burning in the middle of the science lab. It had been thin and colorful and although hot, he wanted to touch it – to see how scorching it really was. The flame from that erupting combustion had quickly spread upward, but, as it should, moved more slowly outward. The gas feeding the flame was pure and flowed unabated in a mesmerizing plume that fascinated him. Even though the clean, precious fuel pumped continuously and furiously through the supply tube, the flame remained steady – slicing the invading spring from the opened windows nearby.

Watching Whitestone move his lips as though he were talking, he remembered one of the last days of class before senior holidays leading to graduation. That afternoon in science class, where Whitestone served in his other capacity as chemistry teacher, a gentle breeze entered through the open windows of the brick building, permeating the room with subtle air currents. It was just enough ventilation, not strong enough to bend the flame, but sufficient to prevent stagnation. Stagnant air was never good, never right. He had learned that.

As he ignored Gregory Whitestone that afternoon just as he was doing now, the stream of air from the high school grounds outside whirled around him, preventing the flame from heating the surrounding space to any significant degree. Characteristic of any freely burning blaze, the uninhibited one at his own science lab station had created a rising column of hot, multicolored gases – the beauty of the fire's commanding control paralyzing him just as did every other flame in the room.

Now, sitting in a stuffy auditorium confined in a bulky graduation uniform, an outfit he found meaningless, he thought about that column of beauty in the brick science building – that beautifully mesmerizing burst of fire – and imagined what it could do if not confined to a lab table. Toward the last of the class period, he had reached for the gas handle and turned it slowly, watching the column push higher and become even more alluring.

Had he been able to run his fingers up and down inside the brilliant column, he would have found the fire hottest where the gas erupted from the nozzle to feed it. He knew that. He had already been taught that.

But that evening, a-hole Whitestone was jubilant in his primary capacity with the school, rambling non-stop about how lucky he and the rest should feel to have been students at Larkspur. The privilege of the whole ordeal was nevertheless lost on that lucky student. However, there was a satisfied sense that he had gotten what he needed out of high school, a skill that would become refined with use. The senior chemistry course had indeed been an eye-opener for him, an introduction to a world of fascination that would be magnified by information easily available in cyberspace. He would enjoy being freed from the confines of the private school in Larkspur. Instead he would spend time alone, away from the snobs in his graduating class, remaining out of sight while researching internet sites and reading books, learning to be indiscernible.

The summer following that drawn-out high school graduation was over quickly, an alcoholic blur not just for me but also for most of my Larkspur peers. It started with the annual senior class trip, this time to a palatial resort in Costa Rica. While Granddad footed my hotel bill, airline ticket, and spending money, the chaperoning was left to a brave assortment of parents still alive to show pride in their fresh graduates.

The hotel's amenities were, as we called it, the bomb. As touted on the travel website, there were a multitude of alternatives to getting tan: numerous indoor and outdoor theme areas – disco, fifties, Hawaiian, western – to supplement the swim-up and poolside bars. The movie theaters and tennis courts sounded great, but few planned to use them since liquor was not served. Of course, the girls would thoroughly ransack the high-priced shops laced throughout the resort complex. While the party agenda for the trip was clear, about a third of us unfortunates were still seventeen and, therefore, underage even for a third world location that was rapidly catching up.

With cash in hand, the underage thing was an obstacle overcome by a cell phone call or text message to a kid over in Montclair. The successful tenth grade entrepreneur operated a fake driver's license machine and had become so adept at duplicating even alter-proof documents and hologrammed licenses that his services were also sought by out-of-state customers. The need to be of legal age seemed to have caught a few graduating seniors off guard, particularly some girls. Because of the resulting last minute, end-of-the-school-year flurry of orders for age legitimacy, the greedy kid jacked up his fees but remained so swamped that he never got around to some orders. In true senior spirit, however, the older two-thirds of the class erased the burdens faced by those under eighteen who had been too stupid to prepare in advance. No one was ever allowed to go thirsty except for one dumb kid who spent a couple of nights in the local detention center for an indiscretion committed just beyond the confines of the resort, the details of which were kept quiet by his own parent chaperones.

The must-be-twenty-one casino rule was another complication which seemed inordinately unfair to us. Of course, those who had the deluxe version fake IDs were covered at least to twenty-one, thereby fully escaping the problem as long as an active line of credit remained in place. There were a few of the Larkspur graduates (including me) who were overly prepared, having an assortment of the wallet-sized, laminated ID cards, some of which featured true likenesses paired with earlier birthdates. Other fake IDs displayed uncanny look-alikes with or without different names who had entered the world early enough to guarantee the privileges of adulthood.

A mindless binge of a good time was had by all on that trip, most chaperones included, although I doubt if the parents indulged much in recreational influences other than alcohol. Upon return to Larkspur and after recuperating from Costa Rica, the celebration of life's rite of passage continued. At least for the graduates, and probably for most parents or guardians, the joy of escaping the clutches of the Larkspur Institute for Education was simply too much to contain. Many of my friends' parents owned nice spreads in or around town that were perfect for maintaining a string of unabashed summer celebrations. The blowouts or raves were held repeatedly – all in a commemoration of our years of togetherness, more than twelve for some. The Larkspur police managed to ignore all the summer rowdiness which was generally BYOB or bring-your-own-whatever.

There were lots of late night card games, too, mostly involving the same cluster of boys comfortable in playing with each other. When we occasionally needed an infusion of cash, we would honor an unsuspecting male or sometimes female to play as a moneyed guest. While playing relentlessly, Texas Hold 'Em and the like became easy for me as I learned the craft and method from others. Cards and I seemed to have an affinity for one another, an instinct that would become valuable later.

From a financial standpoint, my grandfather made sure that our family's tragedies did not keep me from any aspect of those rites of passage from high school to college, although I personally hosted none of the summer parties. There simply had been too much sorrow associated with my family for the Foxworth mansion to explode into an atmosphere of revelry. Even though there was a heated pool, a near Olympic-sized one fed by what appeared to be a natural rock waterfall, no one ever mentioned staging a spontaneous, much less planned, rave where I lived. Obviously an understood social dogma was in place to include Sher Foxworth without expecting him to reciprocate.

After graduation and the trip to Costa Rica, my grandfather failed to mention a summer job to me, and I was not stupid enough to suggest one. While a few of my classmates filled custom-designed positions in family businesses, the option of such cushy employment was not available to me. My retired grandfather was the only remaining relative in my immediate family, and there was no ongoing family business left for me to abuse – except that of counting his stock and money market dividends. Maybe I should have approached Granddad's broker and private bank officer about assisting them.

Instead, a typical unemployed day for me that summer began with a return to consciousness at one or two in the afternoon. Once the ensuing party had closed down, my day ended late (or should I say early) with a 3 or 4 a.m. stumble into bed. Like most of the fresh batch of high school alumni residing in and around Larkspur, I failed to savor those fleeting carefree summer days and nights which were predictably hot and humid in the sub-tropical Mississippi climate. But the heat never stopped anybody.

Unavoidably, summer's nocturnal existence was interrupted by the gravity of college. Like most 4.0 GPA high school graduates, I planned to pursue a university curriculum in one of the big three: pre-med, pre-law, or pre-engineering (maybe bio-chemical engineering). Of those, the educational path winding toward medical school lured me because I had difficulty identifying with any other career choice.

Besides, medicine had been a good life for my dad, at least in the beginning, before that girl came along.

Located only a couple of hours away from Larkspur, the University of Mississippi was a fairly easy college choice for me and one that I made early during the course of my high school senior year. Furthermore, I would not be all that far from Granddad, while still allowing the growing room that we both needed. The scholarships at Ole Miss for a high ACT-scoring valedictorian from a smallish Mississippi community gave me a free ride there, allowing a reduction of financial dependency on my wealthy grandfather, even though that issue had never been broached. Maybe the money should have gone to someone more financially deserving, but I had studied hard in high school and from that standpoint felt I deserved it. Maybe I was more worthy of the scholarships from an emotional perspective, a poor kid not by financial status, but because of some other reason. What I had lost was priceless, irreplaceable.

When it was my turn to complete a ritual known as *university orientation,* the time had come to cease summer's frivolity, although temporarily. Not at all particular to Ole Miss, the objective was to live on campus for a few days in the summer, become accustomed to university life before the fall semester started, and battle a computerized class scheduling system. The advent of computers had miraculously replaced a slow-moving, dinosaur method using pencil and paper, or so all of us incoming neophytes were told by our curriculum advisors.

Sitting and staring at the monitor screen in the university registration computer lab, I thought about the boisterous Gregory Whitestone and his words at the still fresh commencement: *superior graduates ... mastering ... challenges.* Taking Whitestone's word for it for a change, I did not flinch. Confidently, I highlighted each of the eighteen hours of science, math, English, sociology, and other liberal arts-type courses that I was required to complete. During each of those two early summer days at Ole Miss orientation, I followed the computer program designed for those involved in the pre-medicine curriculum as the machine led me through registration in preparation for late August classes. Thinking back on it, *led me through registration* is actually too gentle a description. *Dragged me through* is really more appropriate.

The final requirement for my registration in pre-med was signing over the university's scholarship money, which was a mere formality. As I handed the assistant registrar the only real piece of paper involved in the whole registration process, she smiled at me. She knew my intentions for a worthwhile education were indeed admirable and, as I thought at the time, honorable. The few university years ahead of me would be a glorious experience for one as intelligent as I, a mere ritual before medical school snatched me up to continue in my late father's footsteps.

The pleasurable distractions of campus life quickly surfaced that summer at registration and orientation in Oxford. Even for a high school valedictorian, the diversions were not simply indoctrinations but perhaps foreseen. Once each day's computer scheduling, orientation instructional sessions, and campus tours were completed, there was a smorgasbord of undergraduate entertainment awaiting me and everyone else. Most of it was heartily sampled, then left briefly until my official return in late August for the Ole Miss fall semester.

And come back I did, relieved to find the fraternities, their parties and the girls, the beautiful girls, still there, kept warm through summer school. Likewise, the restaurants and bars frequented during my pre-college orientation session beckoned, ready to accept the same fake IDs. Those gatherings that frantically welcomed the new and returning fall students were not limited to the downtown square or the outskirts of the University's host city of Oxford, but as classes got underway, the likes of me were tempted by Memphis, Tunica, and New Orleans and anywhere else within range of a tank of gas. On a few special occasions (and the definition was definitely liberal), one fraternity pledge brother shared his father's private plane and pilot, taking the revelry to another level.

The time spent earning a pounding two-semester hangover at year's end, not to mention memories of morning cactus breath and Visine-proof bloodshot eyes, was certainly regrettable. What was truly unfortunate was that the throbbing, nauseating, and embarrassing headache accompanying a 1.8 grade point average was more than a greasy hamburger, a couple of Diet Cokes, and four Advil could cure. In fact, that ultimate hangover reality had been in the making for the entire time I was at Ole Miss, patiently waiting as the consequence for a derelict, joy-riding freshman who rarely spent moments in the university classroom or library.

The admonishment over my poor scores, principally that from my grandfather (albeit a gentle scolding), was more humiliating for me than the embarrassment hurled by my fraternity in the form of initiation deferment. But the penalty for my immaturity would be the one for the long haul, and I guess my grandfather knew that. Anyone could do the math. The challenge of raising that grade point average comprised another overwhelming hangover.

Pushing that freshman 1.8 GPA toward the seemingly unapproachable and certainly then impossible cumulative 4.0 presented a haunting goal, haunting in that I should have honored my parents and behaved myself and haunting in that I actually did not want to admit defeat. I thought then about how disappointed my father would have been about the whole thing. I still do.

At that point most sane college kids would have dropped out of pre-med, faced the reality, given up – but I just couldn't.

After that wasted freshman year at Ole Miss, Sheridan Foxworth III's liquor consumption was dramatically reduced except for a rare special occasion. Fortunately, my brain, liver, and kidneys were forgiving enough to allow me to limp along through summer school. My lungs were still in excellent shape although the college freshman weight gain made breathing heavier at times. Surprisingly, my grades were good during those weeks of electives, but the leftover 1.8 GPA barely budged.

In the true sense, none of my blown freshman courses were labeled as failures, so the next fall brought me sophomore classification. However, the coursework for improving my GPA during the second year was not contingent upon sop elective courses typically branded with easy A's but rather was loaded with required pre-med science courses: organic chemistry, physics, comparative anatomy, genetics, and biochemistry, to name a few. Whether struggling academically or not, students needing to complete these medical school prerequisites faced the same hurdles, hurdles the medical school admissions department wanted for me and people like me.

Unfortunately, by completion of my senior year, even with higher grades from the non-science courses averaged in, Ole

Miss refused to elevate my academic status to the level befitting a successful medical school entrant. (There was a dearth of bonus points.) Per policy, the university only forgave one *D*, letting me take that one miserable course over – and I did get an *A* on the second go-around.) By May of that final year of university studies, I had racked up a mere 3.16 GPA out of the possible 4.0 cumulative. That's a 3.16 grade point average even with the two *A*'s I got in Bible 101 and 102 my sophomore college year, thanks to Mrs. Gayle for her in-depth teaching of the Old and New Testaments at Larkspur Christian Academy.

While that low *B* pre-med curriculum average certainly did not impress the medical school admissions committee, my less-than-stellar score on the Medical College Admissions Test also failed to win them over. Sadly, the upcoming fall medical school class would not include Sheridan Foxworth III. In the highest degree of futility, I had hoped that by the time I was eligible to apply to the medical school in Jackson, my physical attributes would be in my favor and fill some sort of admissions minority percentage quota: blonde-haired, blue eyed, white boy. Regrettably, my looks did not compensate for my mediocre scholastic record, nor did my family history pull any weight along the lines of *that poor boy, look what his family's been through.*

"Go back and do some graduate work and make some higher grades. Yes, we definitely like to see scholarly maturity. Also you might try a preparatory course or two to pull up that MCAT score," the admissions committee chairman responded when I called him following my final rejection letter. I wish he had just cut out the BS and told me to give up, which would have been kinder. Later after two years of graduate studies in physics and chemistry combined with an additional five thousand dollars spent by my grandfather on my prep courses for the Medical College Admissions Test, I found myself still locked outside of the esteemed halls of the

University of Mississippi School of Medicine. And there I was, twenty-four years old and never having brought home a paycheck except for the summer after the eleventh grade when I sat as Larkspur Country Club lifeguard.

On the other hand, that circumstance would soon change, if only minimally. Not that becoming a high school teacher and improving the education of America's youth does not demand a degree of respect; it surely does. It's just not a big money-maker, particularly when returning to teach biology, physics, and chemistry, of all things, under the auspices of the ever-present Mr. Gregory Whitestone. Strangely enough, I landed that position in mid-August after completing graduate school when another delighted young man was suddenly elevated into the upcoming freshman medical school class at the University of Mississippi – the same class that was missing Sheridan Foxworth III.

Actually, I owe that first steady job to my grandfather and his old-crony networking. While leading his weekly Thursday afternoon golf foursome at the Larkspur Country Club and ignoring the Mississippi summer heat and humidity, the most senior Sheridan Foxworth learned of the unexpected private school faculty opening. The news broke by way of an inopportune cell phone call received by another golfer shortly before my grandfather's eighth hole tee off.

"Lin, we have an understanding about those things out here," he chided his longtime golfing partner, Linton Desselle. "You could've at least kept it on vibrate!" he added gruffly but still playfully as he delayed his swing. Checking the caller ID on the phone display, Desselle grinned widely, then walked near the adjoining pines and magnolias to take the call.

Taking for granted that his buddies would be as thrilled as he, the exuberant Linton Desselle soon bolted from the grove of trees to drop his news on my grandfather and the other two men of the foursome. "My grandson Oby just got a call from the medical school in Jackson. He's been accepted for the fall semester, but he actually starts later this month. We've got to get him an apartment down there as soon as possible. You know how my daughter is. Charlotte'll go all out fixin' it up. I'm so proud of Oby. I knew he could do it!"

"Lin, wasn't your grandson supposed to teach science at the institute this fall?" one of the other men inquired, forcing genuine interest while igniting my grandfather's thought processes toward his own grandson. As his brain and stomach churned simultaneously, Granddad worked toward suppressing the natural human twinge of jealousy.

"Yeah, all year long that Whitestone fellow's been bugging the hell out of Oby to teach high school science for him, but my son and his wife really thought Oby would get into med school this time. Of all their kids, he's always made the best grades. Well, it was May, and he still hadn't gotten in the fall class. We were all real surprised, you know, with his grades being so good and everything, particularly with that last MCAT score he made."

Ever the gentleman, my grandfather listened patiently while delaying his tee-off and keeping each jealous bone flexible. Noticing that a foursome was crossing the stone bridge over the water hazard surrounding the last green and rapidly playing up behind them, he interrupted the gloating grandfather. "Lin, we really need to keep ... "

Deselle had become oblivious to their game and a growing aggravation to his other three regular partners. "We really thought our boy would have been accepted to that med school in Jackson a lot sooner than this. Nobody really understood the delay, even his professors at Georgia." My granddad tightened the grip on his three wood. "Anyway, he's such a smart kid and really didn't need to be wasting those talents. I told him to go ahead and sign a contract with Whitestone and teach those deserving kids."

Granddad's grip tightened further along with his jaw muscles as he adjusted his stance and looked itchingly toward the distant flag. "The whole family has kept its fingers crossed this past week," Deselle elaborated. "This past Monday Oby heard through the grapevine that the guy above him on the alternate acceptance list had gotten in — some kid from Gulfport. Learning that, he thought he might get the same. So for the last several days, the whole family has felt it just a matter of time. Yep, my boy just got 'thumbs up.' "

With that, my grandfather's shot landed on the green of the par four hole. "I'm sure Greg Whitestone will understand," Granddad commented as he smiled both in reference to his ball's placement and the headmaster's sudden loss of a high school science teacher. "Let's move along," he urged as he walked over to his electric cart. "That group behind us is breathing down our necks."

"Well, Gregory will just have to understand. My grandson shouldn't waste his intelligence teaching school. Regardless of any contract he has signed with Whitestone's people, that's just not the way for my grandson to grow socially or academically," Desselle shrugged. He tastelessly did not know when to shut up, or maybe he didn't care. At that moment old man Desselle was beaming to such a degree that late night golf would have been possible had the game run over. His boisterous attitude over his grandson's achievement shamelessly overrode the embarrassment he should have felt for his longtime golfing friend, a dear friend whose own grandson had still been overlooked by the medical school. If there had been any feeling of awkwardness on Mr. Desselle's behalf, he easily camouflaged it. Still pressing the issue as they all moved along the cart path toward the green, he decided, "I'm sure Oby can get out of this teaching thing. I'll call Whitestone from the Nineteenth Hole as soon as we finish."

Even as Oby's grandfather continued to mutter to himself,

my grandfather made a smooth, accurate putt into the cup of number eight as he planned to get in touch with me as soon as the game concluded. Since he believed there was no hope for his own grandson to be plucked from a miserable spot deep down on the medical school alternate list, he wanted to line me up for the newly available teaching slot. After shooting an eagle on the next hole and further pondering his longtime golf partner's good news, Granddad Foxworth decided to call me on the club phone mounted behind a thicket of nearby pampas grass. Before teeing off from number 10, he strongly recommended that I apply immediately for the lucky young Desselle's vacated teaching job. There was no argument.

Denying my own jealousy over Oby Desselle's great news would have been contrary to human nature. Upon getting the directive call from Senior, I sat back in my student house in Oxford, Mississippi, relaxing in a worn, heavily-stuffed leather chair that was a hand-me-down from my grandfather. Long ago he had replaced the piece with something much finer. I thought about the fact that a smiling Oby Desselle would soon be rubbing elbows with the rank and file of the next gross anatomy and histology labs, soaking up the smell of formaldehyde.

"Good for him, the bastard!" I remember shouting aloud during a solitary toast with whatever type of longneck beer I was drinking at the time. Remember, I had minimized my consumption of alcohol, but was far from dry. "Good ole Oby Desselle. The freak stayed in the running for medical school and eventually conquered the system; the boy never gave up, like my grandfather thinks I should. A damn high school science teacher! Shit!" I recalled shouting to the deer head mounted on the wall across the room as I unscrewed another bottle in the spirit of my freshman undergraduate year and threw the top at the trophy.

"That asshole made it. Aha! Succeeded where I failed – where I lost the game. Here's to you and your stinking, rotting cadaver, Oby," I toasted. "Fuck you both!" I added as the fourth longneck went down quickly.

Without hesitation, the desperate headmaster hired me, filling his teaching void and sparing me another year of postgraduate university classes and MCAT preparation courses. After all, I needed a break from my ill-fated pursuit of a career in medicine.

Despite the fact that signing on as an educator was primarily an attempt to pacify my grandfather, I soon recognized the satisfaction of teaching kids with less grasp of the sciences than I. While I certainly never intended classroom instruction as a long-term career goal, Granddad had been wise to steer me to a job more constructive than drinking beer and playing pool.

However, after several months at my high school alma mater of grading papers, taking up tickets at various athletic events, and spending long hours at night on the telephone with concerned parents, I reached an inevitable conclusion regarding the slim teaching salary. The magnitude of its dead-end absurdity peaked one late evening after an hour-long telephone conversation with the desperate mother of a hopeless student, a shapely daughter with an unbending *F* in classroom biology. While at that moment I did decide to rescue myself from educator's prison and give the MCAT one last try on the upcoming spring testing date, I was disappointed in the resulting score despite completing an on-line review course. Then I realized with clarity that Sheridan Foxworth III was drowning and needed to make different occupational arrangements.

And I did, or maybe everyone I touched made me.

Gulf Shores Drive is the main thoroughfare for Holiday Isle, a strip of condominium complexes mixed with spacious beachfront homes that survived the latest hurricane. Basically only a two-lane paved road, the drive is well-traveled for a section of Destin, Florida, that never sleeps as it terminates in a series of cul-de-sacs lined with pastel-colored yet radiant row houses. Each of the expensive dwellings consists of several stories that seem to rise magically from the marshes of the peninsula. Semi-jogging retirees and young moms strolling babies traverse the well-maintained pavement of the neighborhood which is bordered during most of the year by red tropical blooming plants. To complete the ambience of Holiday Isle, celebrating high school and college students reemerge on late afternoons from hotel cocoons to swarm the beaches as a rowdy insomniac herd.

Heading west on Gulf Shores Drive to reach the pricey, pastel homes in the cul-de-sacs of Holiday Isle, one passes a single story compound of diminutive apartments placed on the non-beachfront side, dwellings so nondescript that the strolling vacationer would assume them to be storage sheds. Much to the disappointment of Wayne Simmons, his low-priced rental within this row of plain white buildings did not even back up to the series of canals crossing the bay area between Gulf Shore Drive and Emerald Coast Parkway. Since his most recent client had been skimpy on requested services, Wayne was low on expendable funds, having been forced to settle for a lower fee for a simpler job.

Smaller fee for smaller service: a motto appropriate for any businessman, specifically one who worked on referral. Nevertheless, the project had been completed successfully and with great stealth, leaving authorities stupefied – an invisible trademark for Wayne Simmons.

Chapter
2
•••
THE LETTER

"Whaddaya mean you ain't coming back next year?" the headmaster instinctively reverted to his upbringing, to a time before receiving his Doctorate in Education. "I know ya still haven't been accepted to medical school because Mr. Foxworth, your grandfather, would've told me at our last school board meeting."

"Thanks for rubbing it in," I almost responded. Instead I remembered my Foxworth upbringing and stretched. "Mr. Whitestone, this opportunity to teach science here, particularly under you as department head, has not gone unappreciated. I have definitely enjoyed being around the kids, but a career in education was not what I planned. Of course, the fact that I don't even have a teacher's license has never been addressed."

"Oh, don't worry about that for now. As long as we show our friends at the Mississippi Academy of Private Schools that we had to hire you as a last resort, then we can limp along for a few years without your being fully licensed."

"Fully licensed? I'm not licensed at all and have no plans to be, Mr. Whitest … "

"Please call me Greg. And you could just take some more education classes along, working to qualify for a teaching certificate."

"Mr. Whitestone, uhh, Greg, I never took one education course at Ole Miss ... " (The Education Room that I frequented in college was not the one with the professors, desks, and laptops – even though on Thursday nights I did spot several of the teachers in the cleverly named bar partying right there beside me.) " ... and don't plan to."

"Son, you just go on over to Cleveland and enroll in night school at Delta State. It won't take a smart fellow like you long to get that certificate. I'll bet your grandfather will pay for the classes." Gregory Whitestone's grammar and demeanor had turned polished. "As long as we can show those guys down in Jackson that a dedicated boy like you is working toward a teaching degree ... "

Being called *son* by someone outside my immediate family has always irked me, and no one over twenty-one wants to be called *boy*. Interrupting his attempted ingratiation and choosing not to call him *Greg*, I explained, "You're missing my point, Mr. Whitestone. It's not that teaching's not an admirable and worthwhile occupation, because it is. It's just that I need to look ahead. My calling is something else other than that of schoolteacher, I'm afraid."

"Look, Son, you have done a bang-up job here during this school year. The kids all seem to like you, and several of the parents here at Larkspur Institute have called to comment on your work, quite favorably, I might add."

He was stretching, and we both knew it.

"Some of our patrons tell me that their kids have done their best science coursework ever under you. And that includes when I've taught them!" he struggled.

Resisting his almost pleading green eyes, I strove to block any thoughts of enjoyable aspects of my first teaching year. Most memorable was the flirting from some of the junior and senior girls that was as flattering as it was almost humorous. That special attention toward me was quickly circumvented, more out of precaution than for any other reason. The last thing I needed were accusations of impropriety with minors in the classroom or elsewhere – the final blemish on a record of unimpressive recent accomplishments.

The point I wanted to get across to Gregory Whitestone, but lacked the tact to make, was that I could not settle for a teacher's salary regardless of my grandfather's wealth, not for the long term or even the short term. Throughout the year Whitestone's help to me in organizing the science curriculum for my classes had been invaluable, and I did not want to insult him. After all, he had made secondary education his career. No doubt he would attempt to argue away my concern about low classroom instructor pay with offers of extra work, like coaching some sport or teaching driver's education to justify a higher salary. He might even suggest something ridiculous like following the lead of several of the school's coaches and farming the fertile terrain of the nearby Mississippi Delta, some years with financial success. I simply could not picture myself running down a basketball court holding a clipboard or having to drive a tractor in near hundred-degree humidity before going home to grade papers. There had to be an alternative.

What I wanted to explain to good ole Greg was what I believed he already understood. By default, I had arrived at this lofty station of life as a high school science teacher. The position fell to me, or on me, as the result of a rejection by someone who had achieved where I had failed. There was no question that acceptance of this low-paying job was at the emphatic suggestion

of my sole grandparent, with whom I maintained an emotional
tie that extended beyond mere familial respect. When Granddad
had relayed the teaching opportunity to me from his unofficial
employment service perched at the Larkspur Country Club Golf
Course, I felt certain that he was genuinely interested in my
success and my happiness.

As thoughts of the Foxworth backup money clanged in
Whitestone's mind, he mentally refuted my unspoken concern
over meager schoolteacher wages. *"He couldn't be worried
about needing any money. No tellin' what kinda trust fund
Foxworth has set up for him. The old guy just wants to keep his
grandson busy doing something 'sides chasin' women."* Initially
in challenging my decision not to return to teaching science the
next year, the school headmaster was professional enough not to
broach the subject of my presumed inheritance.

Like Gregory Whitestone and most of the community, I had
assumed that the elder Sheridan Smith Foxworth had arranged
some sort of trust fund for me, although I never inquired
about any potential inheritance. Regardless of my late father's
accomplished medical career, there was not much left in my
parents' estate at their deaths, except for my education savings
and the dregs of Dad's retirement fund. Both funds were fairly
depleted: the education fund drained by my extended schooling,
coupled with repeated tuition for medical school admission prep
courses, while the equity of the retirement fund dove with turn-of-
the-century stock corrections.

"If you're worried about money, Son, I'm sure that your
grandfather is going to take care of you," the headmaster
commented, changing direction while pushing the boundary of
persuasion.

Bristling somewhat, but trying not to take offense at the personal reference, I pushed forward with my resignation and handed him the prepared formal letter. "Thank you for the opportunity here, Mr. Whitestone. I have fulfilled the stipulation in my contract by giving the required notice. Of course, I will complete the present term through exams." Shaking my hand as I left his office, the headmaster looked down in defeat, or maybe disgust, rolling his eyes in a head moving slowly from side to side. Simultaneously he tossed my neatly typed letter into a tray atop his mahogany desk.

The rest of the academic year flew by. The junior classes voiced their regret that I would not be staying to teach them as seniors. I even got a few calls and notes from parents asking me to reconsider my departure from their school. Those efforts seemed sincere, but I still suspected that many originated as plots from Whitestone's office.

What I did find smooth were the references made toward me in the end-of-the-school-year senior comedy skits. I especially appreciated the fact that the senior boy who played me in one satire was the star quarterback who had just been chosen Most Handsome and Most Likely to Succeed. The female actresses playing themselves swooned when he walked on stage into my make-believe classroom. Another sketch bordered on censure. This time the first runner-up in the pretty-boy contest portrayed yours truly in a role that associated my departure from school teaching with my coming under the wing of a 'sugga momma,' amply cast in the comedy routine by the Most Beautiful winner. While the post-performance comments of my fellow instructors hinted at their jealousy, I noticed one teacher laugh until his hairpiece slipped.

Even though my monthly teacher's salary was depressing, I had kept my overhead low in parallel, creating a positive year-end checking account balance. Opportunely, the school system paid its teachers and coaches on a calendar year basis, preventing destitution for me throughout the following unemployed summer. Had that twelve month salary system not been in place, I would still have had two other financial resources as a cushion.

First, there was the rental income from the house I had vacated in Oxford after my six-years of education there, two years longer than planned. Of course, when my grandfather purchased the place for me at the end of my freshman year, it was not for a job well done, but for investment purposes. While he chose real estate over room rent, most guardians would have stuck dependents like me in a old dorm located as close to the study cubicles of the library and as far from alcohol as possible. But he did not; maybe he believed there was still promise for his bloodline. Because of what had happened to my mother and father, Granddad had decided to title the house in my name. Consequently, without a lien on the fourteen hundred square-foot, two bedroom bungalow, the house had considerable equity, a second potential financial resource should I need one.

Fortunately, the escalation of the real estate values and the demand for conveniently located rental property in Oxford continued past the Eli Manning football dynasty and even applied to cozy dumps like mine off South Lamar Street. A couple of Ole Miss fraternity brothers attending law school succeeded me, inhabiting the house to keep the rent checks coming regularly, easily offsetting my own housing expenses in Larkspur. Even without solicitation, the guys exercised their option for a twelve-month lease renewal just as I quit Greg Whitestone.

Therefore, since I had housing, grocery, and beer money, there was no immediate internal pressure to find another steady job, my income and expenses a relative wash. This laissez faire attitude would have to be short term and could only be successful if my overhead remained minimal, as I did not necessarily emulate

Scrooge but did assume some of his strengths. One method of
capping expenses was to remain unattached, that realization
firmly implanted by the time the high school exam schedule was
completed. As I had packed away the classroom and retrieved
my few personal articles, I thought my financial situation to be
fairly stable – a fortunate thing since the high school skit was
way off base and there was regrettably no real 'sugga momma'
in the picture.

   The waffle house on Interstate 55 stayed open 24 hours and
always had current newspapers in the stands. He had often
considered keeping a scrapbook.

Fire in Five Hills Destroys Manufacturing Plant
Firefighters from Five Hills and surrounding
communities attended a fire at the Livingston Textile
Company last night. Fire investigators from Jackson
are expected here later today to examine the ruins
of one of the city's major employers. According to
the security patrol personnel, the blaze was first
detected shortly after the last shift of workers
left the building around 11 p.m. Initial reports are
that the blaze sprang from the rear of the plant in
the main product storage area. Already spreading
rapidly when local firefighters arrived at the scene,
crews took just under two hours to bring the inferno
under control. Collapse of the fifty-five year old
structure's roof destroyed hope for any salvage of the
building's contents. Shortly before press time, Five
Hills Mayor William Parker made this statement from

the scene: "The investigation of this horrendous fire, a far-reaching tragedy for our community, will take weeks. We are grateful to the Almighty that no one was seriously injured, or worse, killed. But we will get to the bottom of the cause of this devastation."

"They'll never figure it out. They never do," he said as he bit into a chocolate doughnut. "The Almighty couldna seen it comin'." After a few chews he licked the intoxicating, brown icing off his right thumb and forefinger, just in time to prevent it from falling to the table's surface. That would have been a waste.

Then he exchanged the newspaper in his other hand for a mug of hot coffee.

Chapter
3
◆◆◆
THE FAMILY

That Friday afternoon's resignation to Headmaster Whitestone was done in clear conscience, assuring him ample time preceding the end-of-the-year school skits and spring final exams. A replacement would turn up, as always. Equally as certain was a forthcoming e-mail from SSFox on my Blackberry. My seventy-five year old grandfather was techno-savvy to the point of sending e-mail from a desktop computer that still boasted a traditional monitor. Despite his enthusiastic and successful investments in the evolving computer and wireless communication industries, Senior remained saddled with his original, but dependable, Gateway and did little internet surfing or checking of his own received e-mail.

A few weeks before I dropped the bombshell on Whitestone, I had noticed that Sheridan Senior had advanced to carrying his own Blackberry, which I assumed was utilized to track his golf scores and those of his cronies, as well as to communicate. Apparently, Greg Whitestone lost no time in alerting one of the founding, though now retired, members of the Larkspur Institute for Education Board of Trustees – my grandfather.

The rather curt, opinionated response read plainly in the subject list tagged to my new mail messages. The meaning was glaring even without opening the full script:

ssfox@usanow.com ... *What the hell have you done?*

Reading the body of the entire message, I could envision his furious pecking on the keypad, the resulting text composed in complete, correctly spelled words – even including proper caps and punctuation. The gist of it was that as soon as his golf game was over the next morning, there would be a mandatory meeting with him at his house. He wanted to discuss my reckless mistake with me, pronto.

Naturally, I complied.

For as long as anyone could remember, Sheridan Smith Foxworth, Sr., had owned an 8:05 Saturday morning tee time at the Larkspur Country Club that had preceded at least four successive CC golf pros. A major controversy, or better said, a colossal screw-up, occurred a few years prior to my short teaching career during computerization of the pro shop golfing schedule and business records. The secretary, who promptly became the former secretary, failed to copy most of the golf course scheduling information to the files of the updated computer program. The recipient of the ex-secretary's blunder was a new member, an unsuspecting pharmaceutical salesman exercising a perk of his recently acquired job. Regrettably, he accepted the coveted tee time.

The furor that ensued was not personally witnessed by me, but the tale has often been fodder for cocktail and dinner parties, no doubt with increasing embellishment at each rendering. Four men in their late sixties and early seventies, led by a thin, six-foot-two gentleman with a full head of thick gray hair, nearly came to physical blows with four guys in their late twenties over which group had the rights to the early tee time. One of the competing younger guys threw out his back posturing, while Oby Desselle's grandfather feigned a near heart attack. The tense situation was compounded by the backlog of other golfers, lining up angrily behind the sudden, unlikely eightsome. The lengthy line of loaded golf carts multiplied along the cart path, made worse by other double booking errors.

From an enormous picture window which overlooked the lush course from his office, the golf pro eventually spotted the escalating fiasco. A gift certificate for golf lessons, gratis country club meals, and on-the-house pro shop merchandise persuaded the salesman and his group to acquiesce to the more mature, angry gentleman and his likewise annoyed associates. Consequently, traffic resumed along the fairway and the golf professional retained his job. The freshman foursome played later in the day with the pro and one of the assistants following along as coaches.

Needless to say, along with the rest of Larkspur, I have since remained aware of Granddad's standing Saturday tee time. Understanding full well that his perception of my career predicament was not going to interrupt his golf game, I waited until four o'clock to drive over to his house. I had hoped that eight hours would have given the old man plenty of time to complete his round and get a whiskey and popcorn buzz from The Nineteenth Hole.

My grandfather presided in an imposing house in a neighborhood he established in the late 1940s. Along with two other developers, they capitalized on the area's topography, the abrupt junction of the Mississippi Delta flatlands with the rolling hills of north central Mississippi. Many of the multi-acre plots of land within the neighborhood encompassed both geographical distinctions. In 1948 Sheridan S. Foxworth chose one of the more desirable of those parcels to build a home for his new wife and their prospective only child, my father.

Following its completion in 1951, the expansive traditional, three-story brick mansion was the largest ever designed and constructed in Larkspur. The achievement would go unchallenged until decades later. However, the only two homes that initially rivaled my grandfather's in their Manorwood Heights Subdivision were the two his business partners soon constructed in the much sought-after residential development. Along with the manors erected by the other builders, my grandfather's home was one of those striking, picture-perfect structures routinely included in the city tours or repeatedly put on exhibition for worthwhile charity fundraisers.

By Mississippi standards the financial success of my grandfather and the other two commercial entrepreneurs was unprecedented for the era, unprecedented but facilitated by good timing. All three men were of a generation poised to capitalize on the lumber and building booms generated by American postwar expansion. A lot of the raw materials required for that growth were produced by the dense pine forests of the southeastern section of the United States, many of which the three men had acquired.

Through shrewd investments and various opportunistic business dealings, Sheridan Smith Foxworth and his associates accumulated a substantial share of the property that was to produce those building materials. Land owners and other financial concerns that never recovered from the Great Depression were easy takeover targets for the trio as they churned real estate profits into more acquisitions, all masterminded by the genius of my soon-to-be extremely wealthy grandfather.

Now about a half century later, I passed through the entrance gates leading to my grandfather's house. After turning off Foxworth Road with definite apprehension and ascending the hilly, curvaceous drive toward the main entrance, I struggled mentally for additional arguments supporting my stance. In contrast to my increasing nervousness over confronting the master of the estate, the lavender and pinkish red azaleas that had lined the fifty year-old driveway bloomed bravely and with great vitality against a backdrop of pink and white dogwoods. My grandmother had been an avid gardener and self-taught landscape architect. When her health failed and she permanently left the house, my grandfather feigned interest in her pristine grounds by employing a horticultural staff. As a result of the fulltime maintenance, the gardens and surrounding turf were so immaculate that, not knowing better, one would have guessed that Mrs. Sheridan Foxworth, Sr., was still in supervision.

Pulling up to the house in my Jag, I hesitated in front of the tall, thick mahogany doors of the main entrance, a familiar but nevertheless imposing sight. I thought about my father's growing up in that house, that enormous, overpowering brick building, covered in fig vine and draped by ancient oaks. His boyhood bedroom was the one to the far left, on the side of the house near the pool. After Dad graduated from the former Larkspur Christian Academy, my grandparents left his room untouched, his entire stash of treasured football and baseball trophies on display.

Whenever I went over there as a child, I would sneak away to sit alone in the deep leather chair still resting in the center of Dad's large bay window. For some reason I equated that roomy, soft, masculine chair with being a doctor. I guess it was because Dad had mentioned to me once that he used to come home from the university on weekends, prop there in that chair to devote endless hours studying his science and math courses, mastering the prerequisites for medical school.

Another reason my father's original bedroom remained relatively untouched was that even after he, my mom, and I moved in with

Granddad, we lived in the adjoining pool house rather than in the main residence. The two spacious bedrooms with adjacent marble-covered bathrooms, fully equipped kitchen, lounging porch, and expansive living area with stone fireplace were certainly not roughing it by any standard. During the ten months my parents spent in that roomy, luxurious poolhouse, which easily qualified as a permanent guesthouse, they seemed perfectly comfortable.

That was the last place they lived.

When I was in elementary school, I used to take advantage of still safe and secure Larkspur by bicycling in front of my grandparents' house on the way home. Even though located just outside the city limits, what we still called an academy stood in fairly close proximity to our neighborhood and that of my grandparents. While weaving in and out of traffic or crossing intersections as I jumped from sidewalk to sidewalk during each afternoon bicycle ride, I never felt unsafe or unsheltered as my grandmother waited for me after school.

She would unsurprisingly act surprised every afternoon when I stopped by. "Oh, Sher, you've come to see Memaw! I think I may have some fresh cookies. Yes, Chrissie just might have baked some today!"

Of course, her housekeeper of thirty-eight years had baked at least a dozen soft, chewy, still-warm cookies just as she had done each afternoon between two thirty and three since my father was small. Generally, the irresistible creations were chocolate chip, sometimes oatmeal, occasionally sugar or macadamia nut. I never knew how old Chrissie Funchess, the cook, was then and still don't, but I always assumed that she was not far behind my grandmother in age.

Once I hit the seventh grade and became involved in after-school sports practices, stopping by my grandparents' house after school was just not possible. I wrote off my disappointment in the logistics of the time conflicts to the need to grow up, to separate from childish concerns. However, much to my private delight, Memaw continued to supply me with the culinary delights. Delivered to my parents' house after school by grandmother's driver, packages of the soft, delicious treats would be waiting for me nightly after practice. My beautiful mom would pop them into the microwave, so that they tasted warm and fresh. No restaurant, girlfriend, or any other human being has ever made cookies like Chrissie Funchess baked for me.

I'm not sure of the derivation of the title *Memaw,* my salutation for my dignified grandmother, a name used by no one else in our family, particularly since there were no other grandchildren. In contrast, the use of the nickname *Sher* for me was in widespread employment.

Sher. When introducing myself to someone or placing an order over the phone, I have always had to spell it. Occasionally, a seemingly sincere individual pries into the title's origin, a story recanted often enough that I have a fairly concise summary.

The name *Sheridan* was borrowed from my great-grandmother's maiden name and assigned as a surname to my grandfather. His aunt then suggested that he be addressed by *Sheridan.* Then, as the only son, my father scored the name *Sheridan Smith Foxworth, Junior.* Cleverly, his parents called him *Dan* and everyone else followed.

When the Third was born, they called me *Sher* and as an infant were careful to keep me dressed in blue. I'm told that for awhile my father referred to me as *Buddy,* and my mother tried *Dan, Jr.* or *D.J.* Gratefully, they never tried *Little Dan* or *Little Sheridan.*

By the time I entered preschool, *Sher* had stuck, and my parents continued to dress me in blue (when not in cowboy attire) while keeping my blonde hair trimmed. Advancing in school, I was naturally the frequent victim of the 'Where is Sonny?' jokes but withstood the ribbing as I excelled in athletics, tolerating the revival of "I Got You Babe" as my own theme song. The minuscule Larkspur Marching Band accompanied the cheerleaders as they sang the Sonny and Cher classic every time I ran out onto the football field. Luckily by the age of fifteen, I had amassed a six-foot two, two-hundred pound frame that offset the feminine connotation of my name – a physique that enabled successful football and basketball careers in upper-level junior high and on through high school. My transition through adolescence with the name *Sher* went as smoothly as possible.

Sadly, Chrissie closed the cookie ovens when I was in high school, shortly after Memaw was confined to an Alzheimer's medical care unit located in a Jackson, Mississippi suburb. Despite Chrissie's support and that of a live-in nurse's aide, my grandfather could no longer manage his wife's disease at home even with all his wealth and the personal attention he provided to my beloved grandmother. The final impetus for Memaw's internment occurred late one weekday afternoon when the police located the once proud, attractive, intelligent, civic leader standing semi-nude in the middle of the Kroger parking lot.

At first Granddad took the private plane two or three times a week to check on her. Of course, the flights were nothing more than misplaced guilt trips over his wife's deteriorating condition and the removal of her from their home, misplaced because she was unaware of both. The few times that I flew down with him to the Alzheimer's unit, emotional though they were, I observed the kindness and patience shown by the specialized nursing staff to my once lovable grandmother. But while Memaw seemed acclimated to her plush surroundings, she would never have known the difference just as she never understood that her only son and daughter-in-law had been killed.

The short air junkets abruptly ceased after my parents' accident mostly because Granddad chose not to replace the plane but then Memaw's condition had deteriorated so rapidly that further visits were just unbearable. Her death a year or so later of aspiration pneumonia actually seemed to bring him relief since enduring the unexpected loss of my parents had been compounded by the agonizing decay of his wife.

DARDEN NORTH, MD
36

Chapter
4
◆◆◆
THE GAME

"How was your game today?"

"I didn't call you over here today to shoot the bull about my golf game," was my grandfather's curt answer that replaced a more customary *Hello*. "Anyway, I shot 73."

There was no further discussion about his golf game. I assumed that the score was shot from the senior tees as usual. Golf was Granddad's only remaining pleasure and had always been a point of personal accomplishment for him, beyond his monetary successes. Nevertheless, the continued disappointment in his only grandson's derailment from steady, honorable employment was obvious in his transparent face. I seriously doubted that today's enviable low golf score had lessened for him the bludgeoning news of my teaching resignation.

"Why in the hell, Sher, did you quit that teaching job? I know it doesn't pay much, but what else have you got to do? You don't even play golf!" Without even looking at me, he threw his hands up as he walked toward the fireplace.

We were conversing in Granddad's library, an imposing room with walnut bookcases filled with antique books that one would never touch unless to polish the colored leather bindings. In the last few years he had added a substantial treadmill to the far corner that was in easy view of a plasma television. His computer was hidden behind a closed paneled alcove on an adjacent wall. Granddad turned to stand before a formal, imposing window constructed of large panes framed in thin tines that showcased the expansive front lawn. It was not until our conversation was over that he looked me in the eye, probably seeing a boy whose accomplishments, as far as he was concerned, had peaked in high school.

When I accepted the science teaching job, I assumed that my grandfather understood that it was temporary: a consolation prize for my disappointment about medical school rejection, albeit a small one. The silence between us was awkward as I broke it. "I just haven't figured out what to do with my life over the longer term." He made no reply. Silence can be painfully humiliating. "Granddad, some parts of teaching were amusing, but overall I didn't really enjoy it."

Senior turned from the window to stare at me, interrupting his study of the front lawn although he had seen nothing but felt plenty. "Sher, I had hoped that perhaps your teaching science would keep your academic mind from shutting down. But it seems you're letting it go, continuing to throw your intelligence away. Guess I should just give up on your going to medical school. All those low grades you made during your freshman year at Ole Miss really pulled you down, destroyed your self-confidence. Of course, you were grieving for your parents – but I was, too, and still am." Weakly his voice trailed off, ending in sad monotone.

Granddad then turned away to redirect his now wet gaze back out the window. His posture stiffened to some extent as his voice regained a measure of vitality. "Foxworths have always been known for their self-confidence. No matter what the bastards throw at us."

No longer able to see my grandfather's eyes, I could still read his thoughts and easily dissect his silence. Even without seeing the pale, distressed face or feeling the lump in his throat, at that moment it became obvious that he was thinking more of my father than me. There was no question that Sheridan Smith Foxworth, Sr., still held immense pride in the accomplishments of his late son.

After graduating from Vanderbilt and finishing medical school at Harvard, Dad completed his plastic surgery residency at Emory. Rumor was that my grandfather's sudden interest in improving the medical library there had landed a training slot for his son, but that was just what it was – rumor. The library received a hefty donation for sure, but Dad would have been accepted to Emory anyway. Despite vigorous recruiting efforts by his physician professors to remain on the teaching staff, Dan Foxworth, my father, broke from Emory after completion of his residency to return home to practice plastic surgery.

Rapidly Dan Foxworth, MD, built one of the most successful cosmetic surgery practices in the Southeast, accumulating a soon-to-be beautiful clientele that stretched beyond Mississippi, encroaching on out-of-state patient populations. The majority of his success stemmed not only from the surgical and clinical skills that produced well-sculpted bodies but also sprouted from his pioneer medical marketing skills. No one in the local region had ever thought to emulate what was being done on the West Coast: provide overnight plush accommodations for plastic surgery patients. It was a financial risk but one that the people loved, whether or not they really needed the body work. Receiving a makeover from Dr. Dan Foxworth became a status symbol, a mark of social or financial success, certainly not a discretionary service for most. The pampering began from the moment the limo picked up the client from home, office, or airport for transport to Dad's ultra-progressive, ultra-expensive cosmetic surgical facility located in good ole Larkspur.

Occupying nearly an entire block of downtown, the Foxworth Center for Cosmetic and Surgical Body Enhancement featured an art deco façade that housed every piece of beautification equipment or wrinkle-removing chemical legally available in the United States. My dad and two other Emory physicians who jumped at the chance to partner with him in the venture sank an even greater chunk into renovating the adjacent, condemned 1920s hotel for their patients. That project included not only renovating and expanding the hotel's rooms into ornate, plush suites but also included transforming and updating the restaurant into four-star quality.

Once perfected, the plush resort, an oasis sprouting within the confines of a small Mississippi town, was connected to the plastic surgery center by a secluded, covered walkway. This convenience allowed patients to check into the hotel and then move back and forth to the plastic surgery center under whatever cloud of secrecy they desired. Those choosing liposuction, breast revision, face sculpting, abdominoplasty, buttocks enhancement, calf implants, or any other physical improvements generally extended their hotel stay along with the number of body procedures, limited only by time and the restraints of bank accounts, if any. As medical and surgical technology advanced, so did the scope of the plastic surgical services offered. Nothing was omitted.

The building complex was configured so that it completely surrounded a courtyard created by razing an adjacent office building. The ownership of that additional property was acquired along with the business deal that purchased the dilapidated hotel and the area for the Foxworth Center. Within the courtyard were a lap pool and a section for private massages and physical therapy. Most of the physical rehabilitation and massage areas were designed to be open-air and only partially covered by colorful canvas similar to that found at beach resorts.

These patient stations were accessible by interlacing smooth stone paths, perfect for an elementary student out for a mischievous bicycle excursion, particularly one high on his grandmother's cookies (courtesy of her maid, Chrissie.) Access to the courtyard was not an issue for Dr. Dan Foxworth's child since most of the security guards knew me and provided special entrance privileges. If I happened upon a rookie employee, entrance to the courtyard was gained by fabricating the need to see Dad about some childhood problem of sorts. Some concocted stories were so outlandish that my successful admittance surprised even the perpetrator.

Once turned loose in the exclusive area, my custom was to sneak up on Chrissie's brother, Germaine, who worked there as a self-taught massage therapist.

"Boy, whatchu doin' in here?" he would say in surprise as I poked my head each time through a separation in the privacy curtain. Great fun was judging whether Germaine or his client screamed louder from the unexpected intrusion. Generally Germaine was the victor, his piercing screams more painful than any of his deep muscle back massages. Because one of those massages was not far from a beating, I was lucky that I never got into trouble as a result of those courtyard pranks. Chrissie once divulged that Germaine secretly enjoyed the attention, and the surprised clients generally forgave the interruption when their masseuse explained that the invader was the darling son of Dr. Foxworth.

As far back as my memory serves, life was good for the Dr. Dan Foxworths. The partnership's surgical practice was booming and even expanded to include two more physicians. My dad became a regular on a weekly local television show that achieved limited area syndication. *The Dr. Dan Show* was a ratings hit, providing cosmetic and healthy lifestyle tips to both women and men and only furthered his notoriety. Regardless of my father's busy professional lifestyle, he still reserved opportunities to join my mother and me on family getaways. Trips taken during Spring Break, Christmas, and summer vacations bounced between such sites as the Bahamas, the Rockies, Europe, and South Africa. Occasionally my parents would invite someone my age to go along with the three of us, an overture which I realize now was to divert me from their romantic plans. As I began to mature in junior high school, I campaigned for my travel companion choices to include the opposite sex, but Dr. and Mrs. Dan Foxworth were not that progressive.

My life as an exuberant student at the Larkspur Christian Academy had every ingredient of an envy-provoking existence: popularity, affluence, and reasonable good looks. However, as I progressed to high school, my father's professional life was beginning to unravel – a disruption for him that would, of course, spread to unstitch the entire Foxworth family.

The devastation began during the latter part of my tenth grade year when that girl, Flowers Ridley, entered Dad's life and mine.

The surrounding customers in the beachfront coffee shop glanced with annoyance at Wayne Simmons' noisy chuckles, then tried to ignore them. The lead paragraph in the newspaper article quoted the area's longtime fire marshal as describing a pattern of unusual burns on the basement concrete floor of a burned-out four-story building. "A needle in a haystack," Simmons summarized stridently enough for the couple sitting nearby to hear. As they turned around briefly, incorrectly assuming that the surly man in the next booth was addressing them, Wayne imagined the fire marshal's flunkies finding scarce fragments of melted electrical wire in the remains. "Those idiots probably thought they were looking for traces of a flammable liquid," he quietly surmised with disdain.

At any rate, the authorities still declared the fiery roast an accident, basing their determination in part on the structure's properly operating electrical distribution box. Wayne laughed even louder when reading the marshal's hypothesis that secondary electrical shorts in the basement caused the multimillion dollar loss. Smiling, he folded the newspaper and reached for his check, thinking about the investigators hopelessly sifting through that enormous pile of ashes left for them on a quiet back street in Mobile, Alabama.

DARDEN NORTH, MD
44

Chapter
5
◆◆◆
THE DOCTOR'S VISIT

Flowers Ridley was the sole daughter of Mrs. Charity Ridley, a well-preserved, demure lady who had a twenty-three year career teaching kindergarten at the First Baptist Church of Larkspur. Moreover, Mrs. Ridley returned to First Baptist every Sunday as a devoted member of the congregation, with Flowers close beside in the sixth pew on the right. Mister Ridley by all accounts had been no-account, and the consensus around town was that his only contribution to the Ridley household was to beget Flowers. Unfortunately, his genes penetrated with dramatic dominance over those of his attractive ex-wife to create in Flowers an unsightly female version of Lester Ridley: five-foot ten, double chin, lengthy hook nose, belt-covering tummy roll, and wide thighs topped off with tubular breasts. The June Allison haircut and adolescent acne did not help either.

Alone in her room each night, the polite, demure, but friendless, girl cried herself to sleep as her mother listened from an adjacent bedroom. Through the thin walls, Mrs. Ridley sobbed quietly in unison with her daughter, living and breathing her offspring's emotional torment. Charity prayerfully fought her desire to

question God of His wisdom to inflict her only child with such
a combination of cosmetic ailments. While she found strength
in her religious doctrine and had fostered in her daughter
that same strong relationship with God, the realization of her
daughter's physical defects was more obvious each year of Flowers'
adolescence and later teenage years. Mrs. Charity Ridley felt
certain that her precious Flowers would lead a happier life if she
had not been born so very homely.

The ballet and yoga classes along with the sessions at a fitness
facility, tanning bed, sauna, makeup artist, and hair stylist resulted
in barely detectable improvements for nineteen-year-old Flowers'
exterior shell. As her mother's kindergarten-teacher salary was
stretched to the hilt, none of the cosmeticians or personal trainers
were able significantly to improve the daughter's unattractive
physical appearance. However, through all the ineffective,
seemingly superfluous efforts toward beauty, her mother remained
convinced that the girl's heart remained in the right place, though
little else on her daughter's body functioned as well.

"How much do you think they can do with twenty thousand
dollars? That's what I've got in my credit union account," Charity
shared with her sister Faith Behneman during their weekly
telephone conversation. Both sisters had unlimited statewide
calling plans, but Charity had no way to burn up her minutes
other than talking to her sister down in Pass Christian. "I'm going
to try to help poor Flowers."

In marked contrast to their plain cousin, Faith Behneman's
two daughters were both strikingly beautiful. Each was a school
celebrity: one an all-star cheerleader and the other, a feature baton
twirler. They both had boyfriends, lots of them. While Charity
suspected that her two nieces were not frequent church goers like
Flowers, she still wished that her own daughter had at least half of
the physical attributes of Faith's girls.

"What are you talking about, Charity?" Faith asked her sister in
the spent minutes.

"I was watching the beauty pageant tonight on TV, and that
plastic surgery clinic was advertised again. There was an article on
their practice two months ago in *Gracious Living* about some new
types of surgeries and treatments that they can do – lots of before
and after pictures, all in color, all success stories – lots of happy,
smiling faces on those girls. You know, Faith, I've been getting
that subscription for more than twelve years. Anyway, I'm going
to take my baby in to see one of those doctors at that clinic. I'll
probably pick one of the older doctors, not real old, but one that
looks experienced enough to know what he's doing. All of their
qualifications were listed in the magazine article, right under
their pictures."

"Oh, I don't know about all that," Faith replied to her sibling
with a genuine tone of concern. "Are you sure that all that surgery
stuff is safe, is okay for your health, and maybe not a little too
extreme?"

Charity resented the comment from her older sister and almost
responded: "That's easy for you to say, Faith. Both of your shapely
daughters, with their teeny-weeny waists and perfect breasts and
teeth, are gorgeous and happy, even if they are heathens and sluts.
But just look at my pitiful, sweet daughter, my Flowers. She's so
God-fearing, but just so tall, overweight and miserable!"

Instead Charity thought better and countered, "The ad says that
all of the doctors there are board certified. I'm not exactly sure
what that means, but I'm sure they are all highly qualified experts
or they wouldn't be spending all this money on advertising. And
their patients – they're so satisfied! They had several testimonials
from some extremely happy, beautiful people, including men."

Not sounding convinced, Faith added, "Please be careful,
Charity. Besides, isn't that credit union money put away for your

retirement?" Through the phone, the older sister could not see the indignant expression on the younger's face.

"I have other funds to fall back on – the church teachers' retirement fund, for instance!" she answered rather bluntly. Of course, she failed to include that her share of the fund comprised only four thousand five hundred dollars.

The telephone conversation ended cordially nonetheless, with lingering, silent uneasiness on Faith's behalf regarding her sister's plans for her only niece. Faith's turn to initiate the next weekly call went unanswered, despite four attempts and her knowledge that Charity had caller ID. It would be three weeks before the sisters would talk again, and the issue of improving Flowers' physical appearance was not broached by either.

During those three weeks, Charity Ridley had pored over the magazine feature extolling the virtues of the Foxworth Center for Cosmetic and Surgical Body Enhancement. For comparison, she even investigated plastic surgeons available in other places like Atlanta or Dallas, besides the physicians more closely available in Jackson or Memphis. However, out of all of those to be had, she confidently chose my father, Dan S. Foxworth, Jr., MD, of Larkspur, Mississippi. When calling the facility's secretary to schedule the initial plastics consultation, Mrs. Ridley eagerly accepted the offer of a private car to transport Flowers and her to the scheduled appointment across town.

The Ridley neighborhood had never seen such when the well-dressed driver picked them up in a black limousine. An equally tailored gentleman in a dark suit cordially greeted the mother and daughter when they were later deposited under the building's porte-cochere. "Please present this card to the clerk at the desk, Miss, when you are ready to leave," the handsome young man said to Charity in what she was sure was a genuine British accent, "and she will summon the driver for your departure." Helping them out of the limo, he then escorted mother and daughter through the stained-glass entrance doors. As the pulse of both nervously quickened, Flowers whispered to her mother that the guy resembled Pierce Brosnan.

After accompanying them into the new patient check-in area, the Brosnan lookalike tipped his hat and motioned the two toward the receptionist. Slowly walking through the entrance into the posh waiting room, the apprehension of both mother and daughter was replaced by awe as they breathed in the appearance of the Foxworth Center for Cosmetic and Surgical Body Enhancement. Charity could just feel her pitiful, unlucky daughter becoming more ravishing by the minute.

As did her mother, Flowers gawked at the intimately designed space, a unique blend of modern and antique furniture spaced among richly upholstered couches and chairs that appeared almost too expensive to sit on. The air was filled with intoxicating, tranquil music delivered by a surround sound system that floated the melody from every wall and furnishing in the room. Live plants adorned every nook and cranny as though the air had been lifted from the tropics and filtered to the perfect temperature.

"It's truly delightful to have you here with us, Mrs. Ridley. I'm Louise, and you must be Flowers," the striking woman purred as she stood at the reception desk to extend a delicately manicured hand. Charity was initially shocked that the woman already knew their names but then realized that they were punctual for the scheduled appointment. "Please excuse me for just a moment," the receptionist added.

As Louise slipped around the nearby corner for some supplemental patient registration forms, Flowers whispered to her mother, "Did you see the size of the ring on that secretary's finger? It looked to me like a real sapphire. With that rock on her hand, I'm surprised she can lift her fingers to type!"

"How could I miss it?" Charity whispered back. "They definitely pay receptionists at this office a lot more than they pay the one at our church. Anyway, I doubt from Louise's face and figure that she has to do a lot of typing." They both had to bite their lips to keep from giggling.

"If one of you will fill out this short form, I'll enter the personal and medical information about Flowers into our computer," Louise continued to purr as she offered the paperwork to Flowers, who handed it off to her mother. Charity then completed the medical history forms, and because Flowers was under twenty-one, signed all the treatment consents. All signatures were taken on an electronic screen similar to that used when processing credit cards in a department store. "To ensure confidentiality, Flowers, we are going to issue you a patient check-in number. We'll call you by this number when the doctor is ready to see you," Louise added as she handed Flowers an embossed card engraved with the number *14* in raised, gold-colored ink.

After the rather painless registration process was completed, the Ridleys were seated in the waiting area to await their meeting with Dr. Foxworth. Charity checked Dad's picture once again as it hung confidently in a gilded frame along with those of the other physicians on a wall near the entrance to the main waiting area. She then turned and walked to the nearest upholstered sofa, finding it to be just as comfortable as it was beautiful. Even though the grandiose building was obviously spacious, the patient seating and reception areas still seemed intimate, private.

Flowers chose an adjacent overstuffed chair with arms so overly soft that they resembled down pillows. Mounted on an adjacent wall within plain view was a flat panel video monitor, transmitting blurbs of information about available body refinishing techniques. On a mahogany cocktail table before them, an immense variety of current fashion, gossip, and celebrity magazines was offered.

Louise had the unofficial title of periodical librarian and took great pride in her job. She enjoyed the perk of getting first look at all the magazines as they arrived in the mail. Before displaying fresh editions for the Foxworth Center's lucky public to enjoy, she occasionally smuggled the interesting ones home for a few days.

"Momma, I'm getting kinda nervous about seeing this doctor. I'm not really sure I want to do this," Flowers leaned over and whispered as she put down the thick copy of *Persona* that she had started to peruse.

Coincidentally, she had picked up the issue detailing celebrities who were thought to have undergone recent plastic surgical procedures. The lengthy piece displayed before and after pictures, ranking the ten best and worst results. Near the last part of the article, one television soap opera star was quoted anonymously, describing the intense pain he had gone through to flatten his abdomen, lift his eyebrows slightly, and firm and lengthen his chin. The written details about the operations were so disturbing that she could not fathom seeing, must less undergoing any of the procedures, no matter how beautiful the results. Overwhelmed with nausea from the surgical specifics that had transformed the actor into a super hunk, Flowers bolted from the stuffing that had encased her, pivoted on the lush carpet, and frantically searched the stylish spaces for the nearest ladies' room.

"Oh, baby, don't worry so much." Charity could sense that her daughter was getting anxious about seeing the doctor although she did not fully understand that the magazine article was the culprit. If Louise, the receptionist and self-appointed center librarian, had screened the periodicals thoroughly, she would have tossed that issue as soon as it was spotted in the incoming mail.

"We're just gonna talk with the doctor for a while and get a few suggestions." As her mother continued, Flowers' tortured face assumed an even more pronounced greenish cast. "I'm told that this Dr. Dan Foxworth is very personable to his patients and an extremely good plastic surgeon, in fact the best. And, Baby, you don't have to get anything done that you don't want to do. We're just here ... " Flowers suddenly spotted the patient restroom area and jumped away from her mother's oration, bounding toward a toilet and relief. Watching her daughter lope across the lobby in ghastly profile, breasts bouncing as they sagged and thighs quivering with cellulite, Charity finished her interrupted explanation with yet more conviction, " ... to see what can be done for you."

"Dr. Foxworth, I need a little freshening."

Darla Bender remained completely clothed as instructed by Dr. Foxworth's nurse. The doctor initially looked at her face, probing as most physicians do as though to read the patient's mind, to unearth those feelings and thoughts that remain hidden even under a cloak of extreme confidentiality. The woman had indeed become a familiar visitor, so much so that if the practice had rewarded patient visits with frequent flyer points, Bender would have already earned free procedures. By that time she would have pocketed at least one gratis breast implant or maybe an eyebrow lift or two. In fact, she had even appeared on *The Dr. Dan Show* in a "Before and After" segment detailing the perfect blepheroplasty he performed for her. Her lips had never looked more succulent. Not only did she publicize Dr. Dan Foxworth's artistry in removing wrinkles and bags from around the eyes, but from the television appearance she also scored free advertising for her real estate sales empire.

Dad had met Darla in college. Much to her disappointment, no physical or emotional intimacy had ever occurred between the two, at least no emotion that Dad ever returned. However, unbeknownst to him there had been near misses. About the time that things were heating up from Darla's perspective, my future parents met each other in a psychology class and things cooled for Darla.

My father had seldom thought of her since university graduation exercises. "Dan, best of luck. I'll be watching to see if things don't work out – you know – for you and Kathleen," she had almost blurted after suddenly emerging from the dense crowd of mingling graduates and family members, robe flowing behind and around her as she moved toward my dad, stealing his attention from his parents. After giving my surprised father her unsolicited hug of goodbye and best wishes, she melted back into the crowd of other former Vanderbilt students, her cap still in place with black tassel swinging in pendulum fashion. "Kathleen had better be good to you, really good," she turned and blasted aloud back toward him, the statement lost within the throngs of tears, other hugs, and true joy.

Coincidence later brought Darla and Mr. Bender to Larkspur, he to become president of the Bank of Larkspur and his wife to establish what would grow into a prosperous and far-reaching real estate company. In the years that followed, childless Darla approached forty but felt twenty and thought she looked seventy. She had become a dynamic individual with stress lines on her forehead, a worry cleft between her eyebrows, and faint wrinkles at the corners of her mouth, a remnant of years of cigarette smoking in high school, at Vanderbilt and later. Her real estate clientele expanded, paralleling the growing patient base of Dan Foxworth, MD.

A true businesswoman at heart, she believed it vital to appear young and energetic, not so much for her husband but for her clients. Changes of makeup and trendy hairstyles had not been enough, though she had experimented with many. In addition, there was only so much that expensive suits and designer dresses and shoes could do in creating the look she wanted and needed. She wanted subtle revisions to her body that were permanent, creative work that was so expertly done that the modifications would create both admiration and guesswork.

Despite being jilted by my dad at Vanderbilt, Darla Bender still sought her would-be boyfriend as a plastic surgeon. All during their one-sided flirtatious undergraduate romance, she had admired his dedication to an education that was sure to lead to success. Clearly, part of the collegiate attraction to him was Darla's certainty that my future father would have a flourishing medical practice and be a damn good doctor.

Mrs. Bender was one of many loyal fans of the respected physicians at the Foxworth Center for Cosmetic and Surgical Body Enhancement; she knew this because those privileged clients liked to talk about their procedures. The plastic surgeon they mentioned most often and with the greatest admiration was indeed Dr. Dan Foxworth. Some of them seemed to delight in calling him *Dr. Dan*, a moniker Darla considered somewhat immature on their behalf. Through an extremely deliberate thought process, secretly comparing the appearances of Foxworth patients to those creations of other mentioned surgeons, Darla Bender made her choice to seek the services of the old college boyfriend who never was.

Seeing no reason to hide from her banker husband the intentions of having plastic surgery, Darla planned anyway for her enhancements to be financed by hefty commissions from the sales of important properties, not the bank president's salary. Therefore, her husband's approval was really unnecessary, although it came easily when Mr. Bender's own informal, confidential research among his financial friends found Dan Foxworth's surgical reputation to be flawless.

Even though Darla Bender brokered the real estate transaction for the seller's agent when Mom and Dad bought their house, Dad had missed personal contact with her at the closing when he was called away for a surgical emergency. Darla was indeed an aggressive salesperson. The hefty commission she garnered from that deal had been plowed back into her looks in the form of removable assets – clothes, jewelry, new haircuts and color, and multiple makeovers – which she believed to be as important to the success of her career as true real estate savvy.

Now she was ready for something permanent: additions, subtractions, tightening, or relaxation – whatever handsome Dan Foxworth, MD, could dream up.

Until the day of Darla's first scheduled appointment with Dad, she had not personally seen him since their Vanderbilt graduation but nonetheless had often thought of him with fond regret and curiosity. She found his doctor face not far from that truly youthful one immortalized in her university yearbook, the one that Darla had studied repeatedly during the years before that initial appointment at the Foxworth Center, mentally adjusting his features for the presumed effects of aging.

On the other hand, when first seeing Bender as a plastics patient, Dad barely remembered her. Cordial and professional as usual, he walked into the consult room for the evaluation, a doctor-patient interaction to be followed by many repeats. Fighting a puzzled look as he approached Darla, he found her already attractive. Sitting fully clothed, propped on a raised chair in the consultation room, she smiled while leaning toward him and issued a businesswoman's handshake. After the reintroduction, Bender crossed her thin right leg over the left as she assumed a semi-reclined position. Her dress terminated high on her smooth thighs, providing him ample opportunity to check for venous varicosities; there were none, not even the tiniest spider vein.

Dr. Dan Foxworth was unsure from a professional cosmetic standpoint that Darla Bender actually needed to be in his office. Throughout the interview, he felt that the patient's deterioration in physical appearance since they had been in college was more self-perceived than objective. While scanning the shape of her face and torso, the lines and curves of her shoulders, bust, and waist, he agreed that maybe she was showing some initial signs of skin excess where the soft tissues along the jaw line were becoming lax and wasted. A mini-facelift would correct this minor jowl formation, he explained – that is, if it bothered her. As for some of the faint lines and creases along her forehead and peri-orbital region, he offered Botox, but suggested she stop smoking before they treated the subtle wrinkles around her mouth.

Approximately thirty minutes after Dr. Foxworth moved into Bender's patient room, number *14* was quietly called by my dad's office nurse. By that time, Flowers had settled her stomach with the aid of a Phenergan tablet supplied from her mother's purse and was feeling a definite buzz from the medication. The nurse led the less anxious teenager and her mother to another area of the building, to a consultation room immediately beside the one Darla Bender had occupied. The mother-daughter duo found the place specifically designated for Dr. Dan Foxworth to see his patients to be even more exquisite than the communal waiting area.

Darla Bender had been discreetly ushered away by the nurse to the check-out area, and the Ridleys never saw her. The Foxworth Center considered it taboo for patients to pass each other in the halls between consultation rooms, preventing the natural tendencies of human curiosity. Moments later, Dad walked into the consultation room, tactfully surveying both Ridleys in simultaneous comparison since he knew they were mother and daughter. Flowers immediately thought the doctor to be attractive, even though older. As she crossed her legs, she decided that he had aged well.

Suddenly, Flowers wished that her mother were nowhere in sight. Of course, her mother was paying for everything that was going to be done, but after all this was her body.

"Hello, Miss Ridley, I'm Dr. Foxworth," he announced to Flowers with automation while greeting her mother with an obligatory nod. He then formally introduced himself to Charity and redirected his attention to the patient herself.

In those few seconds, Flowers reconsidered her initial impression of this Dr. Foxworth, whose cologne reminded her of that worn by one of the male soccer players back at junior college. After a few moments more she confirmed the feeling silently to herself, "Yes, he is kind of hot, even for an old man." She guessed that he was in his mid- to upper forties, obviously tall, slim, but well-built, and certainly smart and skilled, or he would not have made it all the way to become a doctor.

"This is Flowers, my daughter," Charity interjected redundantly in a weak effort to take control of the proceedings. She then extended a hand toward my father as he walked toward the chair on the other side of his impressive dark walnut desk. Behind the doctor's head, just at eye level, she scanned the expensively framed educational certificates – Vanderbilt University, Harvard, Emory University – all awarded to my dad as he progressed from undergraduate school through medical school and to completion of his plastic surgery residency – all with honors. Raised, gold-foil seals adorned other certificates proclaiming Sheridan Smith Foxworth, Jr., as a specialist in one plastic surgical technique after another. Tastefully displayed among the pricey-looking mats and polished wooden frames cuddling the certificates were hung professional photographs and a large oil painting of a smiling, content, well-dressed, rich family of three.

The Ridleys followed Dad's hand signals directing their mesmerizing gaze from the wall decorations to the comfortable chairs positioned in front of his uncluttered desk. As Flowers took her seat, she admired the lush garden to her left, accented in the enormous, crystal-clear window and traversed by stone-paved walkways that were missing the elementary-aged boy and his bike. Flowers would later learn that those passageways beckoned one to the lavish hotel next door.

"Miss Ridley, we are certainly pleased to have an opportunity to visit with you and your mother today. May I call you *Flowers?*" Dad thought back through his years of training and practice and could not recall any previous patient with such a given name.

"Yes, you may, Doctor," her mother interrupted. "And please call me *Charity.*"

Nodding politely in recognition but redirecting the interview toward Flowers Ridley, Dad continued, "What are you interested in having done?"

"I would," Charity almost stuttered correcting herself, "**she** would like to have some changes made to her chin, nose, breasts, tummy, and thighs. I'm sure that you can see that my Flowers is truly a beautiful girl inside, and I want," again Charity faltered, "**she** wants to let that beauty out for the world to appreciate."

"Well, Flowers, that is quite an ambitious plan, all of which we can help you achieve wonderfully," he responded again with an effort not to ignore Mrs. Ridley but to develop a relationship with the actual patient. Concurrent with his verbal interview with the Ridleys, my father's keen eyes probed the outward appearance of this Flowers Ridley. As is easy for an experienced cosmetic plastic surgeon, his quick mental assessments did not require the aid of computer imagery in formulating a modification and enhancement plan for the client.

"What kind of work do you do?" he inquired since occupational history was often helpful to him in meeting a patient's expectations. He particularly wanted to understand a patient's self-perceived need for change and the plans for the body improvements. Dan Foxworth, MD, doubted that Flowers had any aspirations toward a career in pole or lap dancing, but the response to that routine inquiry had often been surprising. Dad had dramatically improved the bodies of all sorts of people from housewives to executives to strippers and suspected call girls. He doubted if this young girl was headed for any one of those careers, believing that even housewife might be a stretch for pitiful Flowers.

Before he initiated any patient treatment, my father felt a responsibility to appreciate someone's true plastic surgery expectations. Through these preoperative interviews, he wanted the client to gain a realistic understanding of the limits of modern plastic surgery as dictated by the products and corrective techniques currently available. And whatever was currently available and plausible was to be had at the Foxworth Center.

"I'm still a student at Venice Junior College," Flowers managed to wedge into the interview with the doctor before her mother beat her to an answer.

"I've looked through the medical history that your mom completed for you," he explained with a repeated nod at Mrs. Ridley, this time adding an appreciative smile, "and you seem to be quite healthy with no medication or chemical allergies. And you take no prescription medications or use any alcohol, tobacco, or any other drugs? Is all this information correct?" After a double affirmative nod from both females, he stood and motioned for the two to follow from the office into an adjacent sparklingly clean examination room. Flowers immediately decided that the lingering scent in the air was Clorox.

The expansive space was adorned with a mechanical chair and

several LCD panels attached to computer software, technology not in widespread use in plastic surgery offices of the time. This computer wizardry would be used to illustrate the physical changes available to Flowers, alterations already diagrammed in her doctor's mind. She immediately noticed that floating across the screens were colorful before-and-after pictures of nameless exuberant men and women, their lives no doubt totally transformed from mundane to fabulous. She tried to hide the excitement she was beginning to share with those ecstatic individuals, truly believing in what this marvelous, sexy doctor and his plastic surgery could accomplish for her.

Cordell Pixler, Esquire, had a new wife, his fourth. This latest matrimonial acquisition was not at all a surprise for the Larkspur social community because Pixler never remained single for long. Anyone who already knew the latest Mrs. Cordell Pixler, or subsequently met her, thought her more attractive and definitely much younger than her attorney husband.

Much to his chagrin, Pixler had not been persuasive enough to coax his voluptuous bride to move permanently into the mortgage-free house, the one his third wife insisted he buy and remodel extensively several years before his third divorce. Even with the 2600 square feet of space added during the remodeling to satisfy the third wife, Rachel Pixler wanted a brand new house. Forget the added media room, master suite, and small but full-service gym; she deserved a home unique to her and not contaminated by the previous, infamous Mrs. Pixler III. Rachel, of course, never had the opportunity to get really acquainted with number three, Sandra Pixler, but thoughtful Cordell had filled in the sordid, evil details.

Anyway, Rachel's ambitious mind required that her own home in Larkspur be a great deal more expansive than Cordell's present house. Furthermore, it would have to be located in the most exclusive area of Larkspur, that being Manorwood Heights. After all, as she accepted that weekend marriage proposal made in New York by an extremely content Cordell Pixler, she made a pact with herself. Her mental accord included having an impressive house, not a mansion, but with plenty of space in which to entertain her friends and get away from Cordell. Mrs. Rachel Pixler needed what she felt she deserved and had pushed for: a unique, enviable address, marking a big dwelling.

"But, Rach, I have checked with three different real estate brokers in Larkspur. There is nothing available in Manorwood Heights, no vacant property at all. I've checked with Damian Robertson, Felicia Davenport, and Darla Bender; they say that no one has listed a home for sale, even unofficially. Also, there are no rumors about anyone selling. The market's just too tight. Since those three are the biggest real estate moguls around this town, I believe they would know."

Cordell could detect a slight quiver in his new bride's lower lip, not a good sign unless they were having sex. "Cordell, I don't care what those three gossips say," Rachel said, with a rising inflection of aggravation. "Besides, all those three know-it-alls do is run around town collecting sales commissions. I heard that on the new tennis team I joined."

"I explained to you, Rachel honey, that none of the property owners in Manorwood Heights are interested in selling. Most of those people are extremely wealthy and settled and just aren't going anywhere. What about moving out to Eagle's Cove? Darla told me about a beautiful four acre lot right on the main lake, not far from the club house."

Rachel was not listening, not even pretending. "There's bound to be something available; I just know it," she declared with a lower lip quiver that now vibrated much too fast. "I took the convertible through Manorwood last week and spotted lots of old houses, ugly ones, sitting up on those hills looking all vacant and lonesome, just rotting away." The quivering had spread to her upper lip. "Damn, they all need to be torn down, just scraped off those beautiful lots!"

Sensing the eruption of an unavoidable and colorful argument, Cordell countered his young bride's exaggeration. "What do you want me to do? Go door-to-door and beg some content homeowner to sell his house to us – someone I, we, don't even know? That's crazy, Rachel!"

The look in the eyes of his sensual yet aggressive wife was affirmative. "Cordell, you are obviously a persuasive lawyer or you wouldn't have been so damn successful." Charismatically altering her demeanor while moving closer to her first husband, she reached up to pull his left ear closer. Almost whispering as she licked the earlobe playfully, she added, "Why don't you see what you can do for me ... for us? We deserve a nice home in that area because you have worked so hard for all those unfortunate people with legal problems."

"I just don't think it's possible right now, not with this market. I think I've done all that I can do, but I'll talk again with Darla. She probably has more contacts than the other brokers," Cordell softened his argument as Rachel began to massage his lower back while pulling closer to him.

"Hobby Dencil can draw off the most beautiful house plans for us; he's the best architect around. It would be a shame to build that masterpiece just anywhere. Our house must be built in a refined, established area like Manorwood Heights, steeped in charm. Places like Eagle's Cove or Raccoon's Peak are not good enough for people like us or our house. And I know you don't want to have to move from this town and mess up your law practice simply to find something that's suitable for me ... I mean us." She moved across the front of Cordell's neck with her tongue, leaving it just moist enough to dampen the inside of his right ear. "Besides, there can't be another place anywhere close that's as prestigious as Manorwood Heights. Don't you agree?" she asked as she pushed her tongue deeper inside his ear. "Don't you want to please me, Cory?"

Standing in the living room of the house perfected for the most recent ex-wife, Cordell Pixler's agile new wife pulled him down on top of her while dragging him over to the couch. Despite Rachel's momentary satisfaction with her surroundings, adequate enough for sex on demand, Attorney Pixler knew he had better give his nubile, youthful wife what she wanted so that he would continue to get what he wanted. He definitely did not want to lose what this girl had to offer and offered often.

Their intimate but elaborate wedding had been months before, as intimate as can be witnessed by five hundred close friends plus Cordell's business associates. Since the nuptials, Rachel had assumed her rightful place as the latest installment in Pixler's colorful marital story. It had not been long since her immediate predecessor, the third Mrs. Pixler, had escaped to Cancun with her massage therapist. Once the divorce and financial settlements were final, the happy ex-Mrs. Pixler left the house and furnishings with Cordell but took plenty of cash, stocks, and bonds along with all her weighty jewelry.

In contrast, the original Mrs. Pixler had not fared nearly as well. Her separation and prompt divorce settlement had been from a poor, struggling Ole Miss law student, poor scholastically as well as financially, but not dumb. She left the marriage as penniless as she had come to it. Even her rightful charge of adultery brought little alimony because the couple's financial reserves were nonexistent. Moreover, Pixler somehow successfully countered her claims, twisting the proceedings entirely in his favor. By convincing the presiding judge that Mrs. Pixler number one had pursued prostitution (despite her horrified objection) to make ends meet for their poverty-stricken household, the gullible umpire practically threw the woman from the courtroom in handcuffs. Cordell perjured himself further, explaining that his then-wife had sunk to that oldest profession even with his unselfish plans to work nights at a convenience store. The final blow to any sympathy for his first wife was leveled when the judge believed that pitiful Cordell was about to flunk out of law school due to marital stress. And, of course, his wife had produced all the stress. Without a law degree, his future earnings were likely to be no more than minimum wage; that is, if he could be employed at all, considering his tumultuous emotional state. Cordell even tossed lack of consortium into his divorce argument since he safely chose not to have sexual relations with a prostitute, even if she was his wife.

As for Mrs. Pixler number two, she abandoned Cordell years later after he had practiced law with some success. When she made a surprise afternoon visit to her husband's office, a quick divorce ensued – one that was definitely lucrative on her behalf. Cordell had little ammunition.

During the unannounced interruption that afternoon, Mrs. Number Two realized that Cordell's private office desk easily supported a couple of prone, semi-dressed, and noisy adult bodies engaged in an apparently uninhibited, rhythmic physical union. Cordell Pixler liked to keep his employees of the female gender and keep them busy.

Rachel Pixler, Mrs. Cordell Pixler IV, had snagged Cordell with similar physical exercises although she was not one of his employees. Evidently she was more highly skilled in sexual persuasion than the former legal secretary, the one who broke in the mahogany partner's desk. A mere salesperson in a jewelry store, Rachel first met her husband-to-be when he was shopping for Number Three. The purchase of a showy diamond and pearl necklace from the appealing store clerk would turn out to be the last anniversary gift that Attorney Pixler would require for his third wife. More importantly for Rachel, her personal delivery of that expensive piece resulted in a sensuous rendezvous with Cordell in a room on the backside of the Larkspur Motor Inn. Mrs. Pixler III was left at home, happily admiring the necklace in her bathroom mirror, dreaming of what new clothing she would purchase to wear with it.

Cordell Pixler's career in the legal world had been as varied as that in romance. After the out-of-state divorce (the especially nasty, expensive one that followed the impromptu desk sex), he was drawn back to Mississippi, where the realm of Mississippi torts was endless at the time. The state's legal opportunities and other litigious enterprises were a potential windfall for an attorney with Cordell Pixler's drive and finesse.

That ambition led to years of financial success as Cordell ultimately settled in the lovely city of Larkspur. First, he sued countless unfortunate automobile and truck drivers who happened to be at the wrong place at the wrong time. Gradually Cordell graduated to the real money. Multiple dentists, physicians, and pharmacies along with the pharmaceutical companies themselves had bankrolled his most recent divorce but had still left him with plenty of resources to start over with Rachel. His triumphant reputation as a trial lawyer had become so renowned that Pixler no longer advertised on billboards, on television, or on the cover of the telephone directory.

The problem with his type of legal maneuverings was that as Larkspur flourished into a rather large community by Mississippi standards, the town maintained a quaint atmosphere – one of those cities where everybody who was anybody was related somehow to everyone else or at least knew everybody else. Because of those cozy relationships, Cordell had for many years confined his visible plaintiff's work to locations separate from Larkspur and its inhabitants. However, by providing expertise to the local attorneys of record, he had served as an invisible partner on some of the Larkspur-area cases, that is, for a substantial cut of the winnings.

Cordell Pixler treasured his position in the social circles of Larkspur. At the country club, at local hunting camps, and in expensive restaurants, he routinely fraternized with a great cross-section of the town's prosperous, with or without a wife. At that time Pixler avoided awkwardness around Larkspurians by not openly suing them or their families, although the carefully selected behind-the-scenes work had netted him substantial sums.

On the contrary, that treasured, fuzzy sense of community was eventually lost on Cordell Pixler, Esquire.

After meeting with my grandfather about my planned departure from my teaching job and before leaving the only remaining Foxworth family home (one could neither count my rental in Oxford nor my Larkspur apartment), I stopped by my dad's childhood bedroom, finding as expected the heavily paneled, wooden door closed. Opening it slowly, the musty air trapped inside seeped into the hall of Granddad's house. I immediately noticed that the leather chair remained resting in the bay window as though mounted to the floor. Dad's sports trophies also stood in prominent position, filling the bookshelves, although their thick, dusty covering could not be missed from across the room. As I entered the almost morbid space, I paused and looked at his bed, last perfectly made by Chrissie and left undisturbed.

Next to the leather chair was my father's desk, which held a few framed photographs of teenage Dan Foxworth and some of his neighborhood friends and school buddies, including a cozy one with Kathleen taken while my parents were dating. Toward the corner of the desk was a picture of my grandparents Foxworth. Picking this one up, I blew away the dust, sneezed uncontrollably, and then read the message written on the cardboard back of the frame:

Congratulations, Son, on your engagement! Your father and I hope that your marriage will be as happy and loving as ours has been. We have always been so proud of you.

Love always, Mom

I made it over to the leather chair and collapsed in the cloud of dust waiting patiently for me, then started bawling.

DARDEN NORTH, MD
68

Chapter
6

◆◆◆

THE DICKENS

Mrs. Ouida Architzel still resided five blocks from my grandfather's house, long after my parents were gone. She and the late Mr. Architzel had been fortunate enough to acquire their estate in the early 1960s as one of the last few pieces of virgin property remaining in Manorwood Heights. Although their three acres bordered on the outskirts of Larkspur's mark of true prosperity and social ranking, the large lot was nevertheless officially within the social confines of Manorwood.

The Architzels had built an impressive, fashionable dwelling for the time, the design of which has been described as *contemporary* by today's standards and maybe *ugly* by some other standards. The house plan was definitely sixties style, with generally eight-foot ceilings except for an indoor atrium located near the entrance. Large, brightly colored ceramic tile prominently emphasized several exterior panels of the house. The home was truly remarkable.

Mr. And Mrs. Architzel had reared six children in that house, all of whom ran from Mississippi years ago with no desire to return. Given that the Architzel clan was originally from Massachusetts, the younger Architzels never sprouted conservative southern roots and departed their bank president father and his wife as soon as they themselves were self-sufficient monetarily. The oldest and youngest progeny still live somewhere in Europe, I think; a couple of female Architzels moved to California; one adult child later died in a race car accident; and another son was rumored to have landed in prison in Washington, D.C.

After rearing the large, unappreciative brood, the Architzels seemed to remain close through the years and were seen attending the Episcopal Church together on a regular basis. Even after retirement, Mr. Architzel continued to personify the lifestyle of a bank president by keeping a regular golf game, although he never played with my grandfather, and never missing Rotary. As their ages advanced, his wife maintained an active interest in the garden club and the local symphony orchestra support organization. Even though the children abandoned their own southern birthright, no one ever questioned that the elder Architzels remained devoted to their community as well as to each other.

As a consequence of that overwhelming marital commitment, widow Architzel never recovered emotionally from her husband's fatal stroke, even after several years of church and neighborly support. A shriveled-up recluse with stooped shoulders and a bent spine ravaged by osteoporosis, she was seldom spotted outdoors, slowly walking her likewise ancient dog up and down the driveway of the rambling, empty contemporary home.

Practically a thoroughfare in itself, Mrs. Architzel's private drive arched up from the street before forming a modest incline. It then curved left to approach her expansive, unsightly home. Nestled among a thicket of mature trees and thick shrubbery, the house rested at almost a right angle to the street below. After her husband died, the appearance of the bulky house began to deteriorate slowly at first, but the downward slide had accelerated during the last few years. Because the dwelling's contemporary design was not bolstered by the day's fashion, its unattractiveness was accented by collapsing shutters, which begged for repair or replacement, and the house trim, which had slipped beyond repainting.

Mrs. Architzel's street was in the direct path leading from that ritzy part of town to my apartment, taking me past her property during every drive to and from my grandfather's. On an early spring Sunday afternoon, during one of the slower excursions by the Architzel estate, I unexpectedly happened upon Mrs. Architzel as she ventured outdoors. Since the top of my convertible was lowered in appreciation of the mild temperature and light breeze, I was able to overhear the elderly woman's weak, though desperate voice.

The calls for her dog were near panic. "Dickens, Dickens."

No answer. No bark from the treasured dog that had been a Christmas present from her late husband long ago.

"Dickens, Dickens. **Dickens**!" the urgency in her summons became more obvious, more pitiful. Just as I began to think that I should slow the car to a stop, introduce myself, and offer help in locating her dog, the small, aged, but still obviously frisky Chinese pug jumped out of a rustling clump of iron plant. Holding a baby rabbit in his mouth, the pet ambled over to his relieved owner and dropped the tiny, limp animal at her feet. Beginning to yelp in repeated high pitches begging for praise, his increasingly feeble jumps were almost in unison with each bark. Since Dickens' short legs kept him from reaching great heights, he could not reach his master's trembling, outstretched, relieved and wrinkled hands.

Mrs. Architzel's fragile stature prevented bending down to meet her pet halfway; therefore, she simply motioned for Dickens to follow back up the drive. "Come on, Dickens, leave that innocent thing alone. Let's go inside." I thought sadly about my own grandmother as the elderly woman walked gingerly back to the front steps of the home's main entrance, her hips anxious to snap with the slightest leg movement. From my street view, the stone steps were a striking contrast: dense and dark as though covered with the green moss of moist shade and little use.

I am convinced that Mrs. Architzel never noticed my watching from the street, just as she didn't realize that I would never see her again.

Dusk was approaching by the time I left my grandfather's house that Saturday, only a few weeks after that poor baby rabbit had met its match in Dickens. The day had been torture in dealing both with my grandfather, as I dropped the teaching resignation bombshell, and in reliving the memories evoked by visiting Dad's old room. I'm sure the afternoon had been overly unpleasant for Granddad as well.

Once recomposed, after having paid respects to my father's memory, I left in my Jaguar convertible, top down, moving along the path that took me again by the decaying Architzel estate. My driving was even more absentminded than usual, causing me almost to veer off the road at one point. So engrossed in regret over the dismal summation of the Foxworth family, my family, I still do not remember the majority of that drive, that is, not until I reached Mrs. Architzel's.

In fact, thoughts about the death of my parents and remembering the loss of my grandmother, coupled with my career disappointments, all produced such depressing daydreaming that I narrowly missed a sharp curve on the approach to Mrs. Architzel's driveway. Fortunately, my slow cruising speed and fast reflexes brought the convertible to an abrupt stop, preventing it from bolting from the curbless road and crushing an expansive bed of springtime President Clay azaleas. Before I could appreciate the preserved beauty of her neighbor's prized deep red blooms, my attention was diverted to a curious orange glow arising from the peak of Architzel hill.

For a moment my mind denied the obvious. Mrs. Architzel's enormous, crumbling, outdated sixties house was on fire!

There were no fire trucks, no police cars, no ambulances – no people milling around watching the blaze or running around screaming with their hands in the air. The surrounding homes with expansive property lines still stood grand, tranquil, almost lofty, among their mature shade trees and shrubs. Those other neighborhood homes were above such worldly, common occurrences as fire. House trailers catch fire; old buildings housing vagrants catch fire. But estates like those in Manorwood Heights were built to be left undisturbed, admired, and protected for eternity. Those seemingly protected structures adjacent to Architzel manor appeared empty that day, not actually serving as real homes, but instead representing decades of late twentieth century wealth. As the orange glow emanating from Architzel Manor spread undeterred to engulf the entire structure, the periphery of the burning property remained calm on that lazy, early Saturday evening, as though no one at all truly lived in the surrounding residences.

Reaching blindly inside my right front pocket, I found no cell phone. Continuing to stare mesmerized at the bonfire above me, my fist next clenched air while grabbing for what should have been my flip phone recharging in its console base. Why on that particular day I left my cell on the apartment kitchen counter next to the refrigerator, I'll never know.

The impulse to call 911 thwarted, my adrenaline surged as I wondered if that lonely, elderly woman was trapped in the burning house with her yappy, elderly dog. Now thinking back about Mrs. Architzel, I'm not sure why I ever questioned that she would be inside, particularly since she had no remaining social existence. Jerking my head around 360 degrees while pushing up in the car seat to resurvey the surrounding area, I again found no sirens, no one running from their fortresses to assist their widowed neighbor.

The convertible's engine was still running, held in place at the curb before the President Clay azaleas by only a foot planted tensely on the brake. I shifted into reverse to pull back onto the main section of the road before curving abruptly into her driveway. Racing up the hill, I reached the front walk of the house in a matter of seconds. From this closer view, it was clear that the fire originated from the back of the site as judged by the thickest section of billowing smoke. Quickly surveying the rest of the façade from the hilltop, the double carport was easily visible to the right, positioned cater-cornered to the main entrance. Within the open air arrangement was a swollen eighties model Cadillac, secure in its bay and likewise decorated with the dust of decay as the vacant slot next to it screamed emptiness.

Bolting from the driver's seat of the convertible, I hurtled rather dramatically over the closed driver's door as though playing a rescue scene in a movie. However, in this drama the star tripped as he landed on a rock-bordered flower bed filled with slick mondo grass. After painfully sliding butt first and backwards a few feet back down the steep driveway, I grabbed the trunk of a mature dogwood tree and quickly righted myself toward the blazing house. Glancing back over my shoulder I was still mystified that no one else had joined the investigation but at the same time was overly relieved not to have shared my clumsy spectacle.

After managing to compose myself enough to run back up the drive leading to her front steps, I screamed, "Mrs. Architzel, Mrs. Architzel, Mrs. Architzel," in growing pitch. The dark greenish-gray stone that climbed toward the main entrance was slippery from ancient fungus and other slimy vegetation. Somehow managing not to trip again as I lumbered toward the front door, my right hand instinctively landed on the doorbell. Feeling foolish for trying to ring the doorbell of a burning house, I next jerked my hand to the doorknob. It was locked, of course, but fortunately not too hot to touch.

My screams for Mrs. Architzel could not have been heard over my pounding on the door, so fierce that the side of my hand began to throb. Suddenly a familiar sound interrupted the beating of the thick, solid, contemporarily-designed wooden barrier: a series of high-pitched yelps coming from the other side.

"Dickens," I blurted as the barking became even more intense and panicky.

Since the front entrance was impassable, I decided on the simplest alternative to entering (or leaving, for that matter) a burning building: break a nearby window. Apparently the architect who designed that house had not envisioned the day when a passerby might need to gain emergency access to his work of art. Regrettably, there were no transoms or windows installed anywhere near the front entrance. My frantic search to get inside heightened as I could hear Dickens's yelping screams reach a level of panic incredible for an animal.

There had to be some windows somewhere. Remembering that from the street view the flames seemed to be coming from the rear, I darted from the main entrance toward the left side of the house, trying to avoid any slippery mold on the stone landing. An overgrown, thorny holly bush prevented access to the first window I reached, provoking a string of curse words that spanned most of my vocabulary. However, the patio was positioned behind another crop of leggy scrubs and, as I hoped, was equipped with full length sliding glass doors to the house.

Even further to the structure's left, a wing jutted ninety

degrees to the rear and was the source of the growing flames. Reflexively, I started coughing, the black smoke almost choking me as it enveloped the entire patio area before spilling out into the enclosed backyard. The wooden fence, which barricaded and defined the property's rear border, kept the area desolate – made all the more so by a fortification of neglected, tree-sized shrubs embedded firmly against the fence.

"What in the hell am I doing?" I remember thinking and surely yelling aloud as well. "Mrs. Architzel! Mrs. Architzel! For God's sake, somebody come help me here!"

No response came, except for Dickens' continued yelps of alarm and fright. Through the long panes of dense glass I could see the small dog now, vainly trying to escape the dense, black smoke that was overtaking the room inside. As expected, this glass door was also locked but like the front one did not feel hot to the touch. Adjacent to the patio stood a stack of leftover firewood, covered by a blanket of rotting pine straw. Grabbing one of the logs off the top layer along with a few slimy slugs, I used the still-solid piece to break through the center of the middle pane. Even considering my stature and level of adrenaline, several blows were required to smash through.

The thick smoke erupted from the shattered opening, engulfing me as my choking intensified. Pulling my Polo shirt off over my head, I used it to cover my mouth and nose but, at the same time, was almost blinded by the heat and opaque fumes. However, in spite of the stifling smoke, Dickens never stopped barking. As I bent to pick him up and get him outside to safety, the dog quickly pulled away from me, snarling between his high-pitched yelps.

"Hey, you damn mutt, this is not the time to take a plug out of somebody, particularly some idiot who's trying to save you!" I swore. Again unsuccessful at grabbing the small pug, I coughed and spurted, "Okay, asshole, have it your way!" as three fingers were nearly severed by a rapid sequence of fierce snaps produced by small, sharp teeth. Nevertheless, the coughing spasms worsened, nearly overpowering me and preventing any further admonishment of the little fellow. Likewise, the density of the smoke continued to amplify, burning my eyes to near zero vision.

Instead of trying to escape to fresh air and safety, Dickens began to literally back away from me, all the while continuing his shrill, panicky bark. The stupidity of my university-educated, science-oriented brain suddenly amazed me. I came to the realization that anyone who has ever seen a "Lassie" rerun or a "Benjy" movie knows that loyal canines lead a rescuer to their troubled master. Through his stubborn resistance of my rescue attempts, Dickens was obviously trying to tell me that his owner was stranded somewhere in the house.

With that insight, I resumed, "Mrs. Architzel! Mrs. Archit …" but the calling was no longer possible without the hot, smoke burning all the way down my throat to the deepest part of my lungs. At that point it was retreat or step forward toward the dog. Appearing relieved, the Lassie-wannabe once more backed slightly away with a look as if to say, "Yes, you stupid idiot. I think you've finally gotten the idea." Dickens then did an about face and bravely ran across the room, disappearing into the thicker smoke billowing from a half-opened door located on a far wall of the den.

Hearing no rescue siren, I realized that all of the heroics had probably taken only a few precious minutes. Some hero I was, I thought to myself: an unemployed science major, not good enough to get into med school, who had further disappointed his only living relative by abandoning honest employment, presently destined to burn to a crisp after breaking into some old lady's house.

Deciding to follow the dog as he scampered away through the opened door from the den and down a corridor to the bedrooms,

I fell to my knees, strangling in the stifling black smoke. The hall space was filled with a pungent aroma, unlike that in the rest of the house, a nauseating sweetish smell. Realizing from the dog's verbal signals that he had turned a corner of the hall, I could no longer see Dickens as I crawled toward the hysterical barks. Soon I reached the loyal animal, who had stopped to wait for me to crawl on his level into what I would later understand was Mrs. Architzel's bedroom.

At the center of the blistering room were the remains of a mahogany four poster bed acquired from an antiques shop in Natchez. I would later discover that it had collapsed in flames, encasing a melting Mrs. Architzel under its searing covers.

Chapter

7

❖❖❖

THE HEROES

They found me wrapped in sweaty soot, breathing shallow
gasps of air, and lying face down just off the patio. Sitting beside
me was the dog, snarling at the fireman who was attempting to
cover my mouth and nose with an oxygen mask. Even now I fail to
remember all the details surrounding my miraculous escape from
the inferno of the Architzel estate. The fire marshal explained that
probably about the time Dickens got me to the master bedroom,
the fire had leaped to the attic and total destruction was imminent.

The Architzel home had paid the ultimate price for having
habitual, packrat inhabitants. Squirreled away in the spacious
attic were completely empty boxes, entire editions of old
newspapers and magazines, as well as thumb-worn paperback and
hardcover novels. Also stored away for an uninterested posterity
were disintegrated piles of newspaper headline and article
clippings pertaining to the Kennedy and King assassinations,
Neil Armstrong's moon walk, and Nixon's resignation, mixed
among printed school awards and trophies recognizing the now
grown, long-absent Architzel children. Adding to the combustible
material were a few tattered quilts and bedspreads used to cover

much of the stored material while mounted deer and boar heads contributed separately to the disaster. The bulk of the items tucked away in the attic was directly above the widow's bed and separated from her by only sheetrock, brittle forty-plus year old insulation, and a crisscross of well-cured wooden four-by fours.

As the member of the Larkspur Fire Department pulled me to my feet and picked up the still yelping Dickens, I looked back toward the house. Although my vision was blurred, there was no mistaking that very little remained of the one story, sprawling residence that had been the pride of Mr. and Mrs. Architzel. An ambulance transported me to Larkspur Memorial, where I passed my emergency room physical examination, completed a required observation period, and then was released to Granddad for a ride home to my place. Unfortunately, my beloved Jag convertible, the high school gift from my grandfather, did not fare as well. Because it was parked with its top down and positioned in close proximity to the house, the upholstery was an easy target for the shower of embers. Loaded with a nearly full gas tank, the vehicle became its own incinerator and practically dissolved in the heat.

For several days, the death of the widow Architzel and the destruction of her vintage home were front page news in *The Larkspur Ledger* before being usurped by the spring successes of the Larkspur Institute for Education championship baseball team. The updates to the fiery tragedy then reappeared later somewhere deep in the community news section. Following the story intensely in the newspaper, I also watched the local news religiously in case the fire investigators released some new information. My interest was vested not only because I had become a sort of local celebrity after the ordeal, but also because I had found the entire investigation of the fire fascinating.

The Ledger's articles did quote me repeatedly regarding my heroic, but fruitless, escapade to save the poor widow Architzel.

The human- and canine-interest readers were captivated by my triumphant rescue of her elderly, endearing pooch. Repeated letters to the editor espoused great relief that precious Dickens had apparently suffered no respiratory or other medical complications from his ordeal. When the heirs declined to take the indestructible Dickens back north with them, many Larkspurians called the newspaper and television stations with offers to adopt the appealing, photogenic pooch. Instead, the family veterinarian first offered him to me. My landlord waived the no-pets rule – anything for a hero – and Dickens moved in with me to occupy a plush, expensive interior dog house. Awarded to the pug by a local pet store, the abode came complete with a free one-year supply of Science Diet dog food.

Published reports from the fire investigation began to overflow a thin scrapbook purchased at Wal-Mart – nothing fancy, but it served the purpose. The first page was filled with a large colored picture of the hero and his future dog, framed in the background ashes of Architzel Manor. The photographer had captured the dynamic duo immediately before the paramedics loaded me into the ambulance and whisked Dickens away to the family vet. An article from *The Larkspur Ledger* appearing on a later page detailed an interview with investigators summarizing the updated discoveries regarding causation.

According to City Fire Marshal Thomas Lisenbe, a fixture within the department and coincidentally the father of my new girlfriend, the sprawling house had been constructed principally of wood and sheetrock, except for the stone walkway leading to the front entrance and around to the brick patio. "It is our understanding that a private fire investigator hired by the homeowner's insurance company has concurred with our findings," he summarized. Drawing upon his personal firefighting and investigative experiences, Fire Marshal Lisenbe concluded with certainty, "The point of origin for the tragic and rapidly spreading blaze was Mrs. Architzel's faulty electric blanket, a potent ignition source."

Never at a loss for words, Lisenbe expounded, "We assume that the single resident of the dwelling was sleeping in her bed and, considering the age of the deceased, was not awakened by the blaze, the smoke, or her dog. Also, the home was never updated to a central fire alarm and security system, much less battery-powered smoke detectors." Thomas Lisenbe failed to comment on Architzel's untimely use of an electric blanket on a fairly warm spring afternoon except in supposing that perhaps she was cold-natured.

Along with the others, that article was mounted proudly in my old-fashioned album. Scanning the newspaper articles regarding the fire and its aftermath into a computer storage file or downloading them off the internet would just not have been the same. Another continuing feature buried deep in an obscure section of the newspaper quoted Lisenbe further: "Chemical analysis of Mrs. Architzel's remains detected no evidence of systemic barbiturates, alcohol, or other drugs which might have rendered her incapacitated. The medical examiner's findings did reveal marked smoke inhalation but no evidence of physical trauma. From other autopsy information, the coroner has not excluded a natural cause of death although the condition of the remains has yielded some inconclusive results." As I scrutinized that newspaper article and envisioned the poor widow's charred, totally disintegrated body covered with seared scraps of bed clothes, I wondered how a forensic pathologist could determine anything definitive from a pile of human tissue mixed with pieces of electric blanket and mahogany.

Ouida Architzel's cause of death was officially listed in county records as *asphyxiation from smoke inhalation*. Much to the local media's disappointment, the medical examiner and other authorities never divulged any evidence of a fractured skull or bullet remnant within Mrs. Architzel's remains, or traces of spilled human blood anywhere in the ashes.

My afternoon experience in the Architzel blaze morphed into a growing curiosity about fire and combustion. Library resource books supplemented by internet websites fed that thirst. When my grandfather heard that I was spending long hours in the library, his comment was predictable. "Sher, if you had spent that much time studying for the Medical College Admissions Test, you might have made what you needed to get into med school."

Other comments were coming at me, but from a different direction. Shortly after the homely Architzel mansion was reduced to no more than crumbled brick scattered among ashes and charred stone, the fire marshal came to visit me twice: the first time while I was being evaluated for smoke inhalation injuries in the hospital observation department, and the second during an afternoon at home in my apartment with Dickens. When Mr. Lisenbe called on me a third time, this time by phone, I questioned his intentions.

As soon as Fire Marshal Lisenbe identified himself, I inquired, "How's the investigation going?" My anxiety was evident despite the forced tone of nonchalance. Of course, I already knew the answer. My curious and thorough research had scrutinized every published investigative detail regarding that horrendous Manorwood Heights fire. The source of my concern over Lisenbe's additional contact was that maybe his investigation had dead ended and that perhaps the desperate fire marshal needed a scapegoat.

"We have combed every inch of the site and determined that the incineration was accidental, but I believe you know that already," he answered quickly.

"Ah ... I beg your pardon?" I forced air through my vocal cords and somehow kept my voice from cracking.

"My daughter, Kaylee, is the assistant librarian at the downtown branch. She mentioned that you've been down there a lot lately, almost daily in fact, and that you two have met."

"Well, yes, sir. I, ahh ... "

"Seems you're obsessed with doing periodical and internet searches on the Architzel case. Kaylee says that you've even made inquiry into similar occurrences on file. I asked my daughter if you had required a good bit of librarian assistance with your ... research, and she said, 'Yes.' " Detecting the playful sarcasm in the marshal's voice along with surprisingly eloquent enunciation, there was no doubting our mutual awareness of his daughter's good looks. No one could argue that Kaylee Lisenbe in any way resembled the stereotype of a female librarian, if one exists.

Listening to her father's comments regarding my time spent in the local library, I recalled the last trip to the public computer bank which fills a corner of the building. Admiring the pretty face that topped Kaylee's shapely body as she helped me unfreeze the computer in front of me, I almost worked up the nerve to ask her to the Starbucks next door. Sadly, by the time I finished working through the topics gathered by the search engine, she had disappeared.

"Well, she is definitely a good ... a great ... librarian. Definitely has made an impression on me, Mr. Lisenbe," I stumbled forward.

"To the contrary, Son, you have made a definite impression on the entire community!" suddenly shifting the conversation away from his pride-and-joy daughter and focusing directly on me. "I've done a little checking up on you, you might say."

Suddenly, I felt guilty, but I wasn't sure of what: guilty because I could have set the fire that killed that poor old lady or guilty because I wanted to sleep with the fire marshal's daughter.

The awkwardness on my end began to grow, but before I could fabricate a reason to get off the phone, he drove home his point. "I heard through the country club grapevine," (I was surprised that the fire marshal of Larkspur, Mississippi, made enough money to belong to the country club), "that you are sort of between jobs or maybe even between careers. Someone told me that while you've been trying to get into medical school you've been killing time teaching science at the institute."

With that I began to wonder how many times my grandfather had discussed my unsuccessful career pursuits in public – likely quite a few. Struck by the vision of Sheridan Smith Foxworth, Sr., randomly commiserating over my plight with his golfing and other country club drinking cronies, I felt confused over the city fire marshal's objective in calling me. Why had the topic of conversation shifted dramatically from the Architzel blaze to my long-term career objectives? Did all of this have to do with a father's mission to become a matchmaker for his daughter, a girl that could certainly take care of herself in the world of romance? Or did I have an exaggerated opinion of myself?

"You seem to be a determined young man, Mr. Foxworth," Fire Marshal Lisenbe continued.

Understanding that I needed to be as friendly as possible to this fellow, I interrupted, "Please call me *Sher*."

"That's what I had heard you went by, but I really wasn't sure," he hesitated somewhat.

Not believing that he thought me homosexual or anything, especially since I had been flirting with his daughter, I explained, "*Sher* is short for a family name."

"Uhhhh, Sher," there was definite hesitation in the salutation as he sounded more serious, "we have several openings in our department, and I wondered if you might be interested."

My bewilderment continued. "Openings in your department? For what?" I wondered aloud to him, confused as to why the fire department needed a good high school science instructor, qualified with almost one year of teaching experience, or a college graduate with four years of drinking experience.

"Firemen!" he responded in a tone that registered shock at my stupidity. "You would start from the ground up, but with your IQ and all you should be able to build a nice career in the fire department."

"But sir, I'm not interested in being a fireman," I responded as respectfully as possible.

"From all your inquiry into the world of pyrogenic sciences, it sounds like you could become interested. Maybe you've always had a subconscious desire to be a fireman and never realized it. You know, it could have begun when you were a little fellow when you pretended to be a fireman."

"Ah, no, sir, I really don't have any desire to ... "

"Well, you, uhh, ... (Thomas Lisenbe still seemed a little hesitant with my name, but I remember thinking at the time that his name was not all that straightforward either)... Sher, you are certainly worthy of a career in firefighting. No doubt about it, the fire training academy in Storck can certify you in no time."

Again I was unsuccessful in trying to interrupt his near dissertation which showed no sign of humor, still no indication that this was a joke or some kind of phone prank.

"I talked to the commander down there in Storck this morning – called him first thing. He confirmed that his program will credit your college work toward the academic part of the preparation, particularly since you have a science background. Once you're out, the starting pay is decent and no doubt you'll be kicked up to lieutenant in no time. Unfortunately, if by chance you had already been to the police academy, then the jump over to firefighting would have been much smoother."

For a moment I wondered if I could actually be a victim of an Ashton Kutcher punk or possibly a Sidney Boykin prank, more likely the Boykin prank since I was not a television or film celebrity. Sid Boykin was a Mu Nu Upsilon with me at Ole Miss. A master of the telephone hoax, even with the advent of caller ID, he practiced his craft at all hours of the day and night, generally targeting those with landlines since those calls were readily put on speakerphone. He particularly relished playing before mixed audiences at fraternity parties as he broadcast the humiliating shenanigans. I had not kept up with Sid but knew that the improbability of his being the caller was as equal to my being punked by Kutcher because Boykin resided in a strict drug treatment center somewhere in Georgia, one which limited outside phone access.

Interrupting my thoughts of MTV episodes as well as Ole Miss, Thomas Lisenbe continued, "Not trying to be too nosy, but do you really need to earn a real salary right now? You know, with the inheritance from your parents and all."

I decided to ignore that comment and tried not to take offense. Clearly, it was obvious that Fire Marshal Lisenbe assumed that I was just some member of the lucky sperm club, having plenty of money but just needing something to occupy his time.

"Every member of our force here in Larkspur admired how you went in to try to save that poor woman and brought her dog out to safety when you realized there was nothing you could do for her. You did all that without any formal training in firefighting and emergency rescue."

"Well, sir, I just did what any ... "

"You've got the physical build for the job and maybe even more brains than needed, but we would really like to have you on our squad. Tomorrow let me call Jerry, Commander Gressett, and tell him you'd like to go down there with me next week to tour his camp. You can meet with him one-on-one about the training required and what you can expect at his facility. From what I have told him about you already, Sher, (the name seemed to be coming to him more easily) he would admit you to the fire academy on the spot and graduate you in no time!"

"Mister – I mean – Marshal Lisenbe, being a firefighter wasn't exactly my career plan. There's never been anyone in my family who's done anything like that."

"Son, firefighting is a noble occupation. Ranks way above police work in my opinion and probably is a lot safer. As a policeman, a guy's probably more likely to get nailed with a bullet than a fireman burned by a two-by-four."

"Well, I wasn't exactly considering police work either."

"Listen, Son, you can't live off your family's money forever. That's just not right. Think about doing something with your life that counts. After all, people seem to look up to a fireman."

"Yeah, if you're a four-year-old," I wanted to say but instead said nothing.

"You'll have to submit to polygraph tests and have a psychological profile drawn up when we go to Storck for the admissions interview, but I'm sure you'll do fine. Kaylee tells me that you're in good physical shape."

I still expected the guy to start laughing any minute, but he never did, particularly after his comments seemed to remain personal in nature and were growing more so. In reality, his daughter had not learned all that much about "my good physical shape," by that time, anyway.

Thanking him profusely for being interested in my welfare, I let the marshal down as politely as possible. I pushed the graciousness to the extreme by extolling him for his own valiant efforts toward protecting the lives and property of the appreciative Larkspur citizens. Hanging up the phone, I got the feeling from his wistful farewell that Fire Marshal Thomas Lisenbe was not finished with me.

Once they were reprinted in regional newspapers, Wayne Simmons read many of the same *Ledger* articles concerning the Architzel fire that I had preserved in my scrapbook. When driving west on I-20 from a job in Jackson, he came across an original print of one of those articles which had earned the newspaper's front page. Some trucker had discarded an original copy of the *The Larkspur Ledger* in the greasy café, which had become a new eatery for Simmons. Wayne read such stories about fire investigations with great delight. "What a bunch of freakin' idiots," Simmons muttered loudly and almost clearly enough for the nearby waitress to hear. At first he failed to notice that his order was ready as she placed the tall stack of bacon-and-syrup smothered pancakes on the service counter.

Mesmerized by the content of the opened newspaper he was studying, he smelled the late morning breakfast as it slid slowly toward him. "What a bunch of damn freakin' idiots!" he repeated with more emphasis, even though the waitress had heard him the first time. Wayne raised the newspaper just high enough off the counter to allow the sliding plate to enter his sanctum as would an automobile moving under a rising garage door. The plate of food stopped against his chest with a swooshing thud, and the aroma filled the space enclosed by his stooped torso, extended arms, and newspaper. Reading on but now folding the newspaper down, Simmons began to laugh uncontrollably while rocking on the counter stool, partially chewed oversized bites of diner food jiggling in his open mouth.

The waitress looked curiously back toward him as she walked to another customer, snatching a glimpse of Simmons' fascination. "You see all types around this dive," she summarized under her breath, shocked that someone would find humorous a newspaper story about house fire and death.

"*Arc mapping, sniff test, secondary electric shorts,* I love it!"
cackled Wayne as he repeated the terms thrown out by Fire
Marshal Lisenbe and his fellow Architzel fire investigators. The
few remaining customers glanced in his direction with annoyance.
"I wonder how much money that old bag had in all," he marveled,
this time under his breath. "*Burn tests, flashover, electro-
kindling,* those guys are full of it!"

"Sir, you need sump'n else?" the waitress returned, this time
with an air of aggravation and his check.

Wayne Simmons looked up blankly at the young, but wrinkled,
woman who reeked of stale cigarette smoke mingled with a
bouquet of pork sausage, fried egg, and grilled cheese sandwich
odors. "They'll never figure out what caused that fire. Never," he
summarized with a grin directed at her puckered nose and mouth,
not bothering with an appropriate answer.

The server forced an even more indignant face as she jerked the
cash off the counter that Simmons tossed at her. Writing him off
as rude, something seldom seen in her customers, the waitress
flipped her head slightly to the right as she quickly swaggered
away, wanting to flip something else. "That dude over there's
got some real issues," she announced to another waitress as she
approached the coffee machine. "But if he'd get his teeth fixed and
wash that smelly grease out of his hair, he wouldn't look half bad."

Chapter
8
♦♦♦
THE TEST

Unlike some twenty-three-year-old girls that I had been out with in Larkspur, Kaylee Lisenbe fortunately did not live with her parents. Following her father's unsuccessful job proposition, this convenience allowed escape of a subsequent face-to-face confrontation with him. The absurdity of that solicitation still had me dumbfounded: me, a fireman.

All the same, during my following "research" visit to the Larkspur Regional Library, I scanned multiple websites and even some books pertaining to careers in firefighting. The facts that Fire Marshal Lisenbe had rattled off when he called regarding training options were correct and to the point. It seemed that qualified policemen could indeed make lateral moves into the pyrotechnical fields with only minor additional training, but then I wasn't a policeman. Among other things, my hours of internet surfing turned up a university in Canada that offered a quickie course on battling fires, complete with gold-leaf framed graduation certificate. I wondered how valuable such a certificate would be in combating a multi-alarm fire in a high-rise. Fortunately, Larkspur was void of skyscrapers.

During the time I spent that day in the library, the degree and subject matter of my concentration wavered dramatically. Jumping from one internet site to another, devouring countless periodicals, my train of thought was so flighty that I frequently found myself on subjects other than pyrogenics such as entertainment news, current events, and historical sports figures; I even played a few games of online poker.

Most of my diversion of the afternoon resulted from Kaylee's multiple jaunts through the research section of the building. Across the aisle from my regularly occupied computer station, she was helping an older gentleman with a genealogy endeavor. While my librarian girlfriend worked as kindly as possible to assist him, the fellow's raised voice secondary to his hearing deficit provided more than anyone cared to know about his quest. The result was an unavoidable exchange at a level much greater than a whisper. "My great niece desires her rightful place in the Daughters of the Colonial Lawyers," I heard him stress as Kaylee worked respectfully to maintain library decorum.

On more than one occasion during his tutoring session, I caught the dried-up pervert glancing away from the computer screen as Kaylee reached down to enter additional information on the keypad. Beginning with her angelic face, his eyes followed Kaylee's curves: tracing her slender neck, through the ample breasts, and along the hips to end at her feet, which were also perfectly proportioned. I'm sure the ancient coot was imagining a genealogical offshoot in which he and the tender but gorgeous librarian would procreate a legacy of their own, or at least go through the motions of it.

At last, the sexy librarian left the disappointed uncle and his exhaustive computer efforts since the pre-revolutionary war lineage was not law-related. As Kaylee nonchalantly glanced my way, I looked up from my page on "The Five Points of Origin" and glared at her blue eyes with a much greater degree of reciprocation. Kaylee seemed to veer casually toward me and put her right hand on the top of my monitor. She practically pivoted in place as she bent down in an apparent *May I help you, sir?* gesture. Masking my excitement, I minimized the research information on my screen and replaced it with this type: *Go out this weekend? With me?*

Bending further to reach my keyboard, Kaylee nearly crushed my face with her filled blouse, forcing me to lean back in my chair so I could breathe. In private I wouldn't have budged an inch, but there in the public library of Larkspur, Mississippi, I felt that every patron was watching us, particularly Boner Gramps across the room. Moving back for air, I read her response: *Sure, when and where? But you don't have a car anymore. It looked like a pile of candle wax in the newspaper picture!!!*

Kaylee underestimated my resources. Well, not really my resources, but those of the insurance company that acted expediently on my behalf. The fiery ordeal at the top of the Architzel hill landed me a brand new ride, all without increasing my insurance rates. Because I was acting as a Good Samaritan when my Jag joined the ashes in the Manorwood Heights fire, my comprehensive loss automobile policy waived all deductible and depreciation clauses. Unsurprisingly, my personal Larkspur insurance agent, who suddenly had become my best friend, was featured in the local newspaper detailing his company's appreciation for hometown heroes like me. The agent's full-length photo accompanied the article that dealt more with the philanthropic efforts of Worldwide Carriers Insurance and its local agents than it did with the tragic death of Ouida Architzel and the total loss of her home.

The automobile insurance company had certainly treated me

right. One benefit to my using such a homegrown agent was that there was no way he could screw over a local hero and not receive a publicity backlash. Although he could not swing an identical replacement for my treasured but used Jaguar, he did team up with the local Ford dealer to substitute a current model Mustang convertible. In fact, once he and the car dealer were ready to make the new car presentation, he arranged another front-page news item about my heroics at the outdated Larkspur estate, along with a color picture of the two smiling businessmen and me closely gracing the prize. No doubt they anticipated much goodwill publicity, all in the name of humanity.

The invitation to Kaylee continued on the monitor screen: *What about dinner at the Rexford? Saturday night? To celebrate my being the hero of Larkspur and not planning to teach again next year. I'll get reservations ...*

She interrupted my keyboard pecking by leaning further down to whisper in my right ear, "Seven-thirty will be just fine. Looking forward to it. I guess you'll find a way to pick me up," Kaylee purred, knowing full well that I had a new car to replace the Jag. She brushed her hips fairly close to my upper back as she turned away, recognizing another library patron near me who seemed to be frustrated over a frozen computer.

The Rexford Hotel remained the only non-subdivided structure within the dissolved Foxworth Center for Cosmetic and Surgical Body Enhancement. The ensuing owners were careful to preserve and even supplement the oriental rugs, oil paintings, chandeliers, and antique books and bookcases that enhanced the building when the assets of my father and his partners were liquidated. Such properties acquired through bankruptcy proceedings are seldom so well-appointed and maintained. While once a plush, yet isolated, recovery facility for the clients of the Foxworth Center, my father's hotel had become the Rexford, a popular (more precisely described as 'swinging') downtown establishment, probably more so for its food and beverage and live musical entertainment than its pillow-top mattresses, although the mattresses were never neglected.

Greeting us at the entrance, the maitre d' obviously recognized me. The slim, youthful, polished man had climbed the ranks from lowly restaurant busboy back when the place was part of my father's business. He took one look at Kaylee Lisenbe and knew that I would want to impress her, that I needed to impress her. Accordingly, the maitre d' seated us at one of the more desirable tables near a window overlooking the gardens that I used to invade and terrorize as a child.

Although the view into the lighted courtyard was breathtaking, the truly intriguing sight was not through the glass but in the other direction, out across the body of the restaurant where there was not an empty seat. The situation was definitely standing room only. Around the bar and conversational spaces exuded a rising hum of merry chit-chat courtesy of Larkspur high society: the stunning people, the rich people. Yes, a lot of talent graced the magnificent establishment that was even more remarkable than in its earlier days. One actively socializing but distinctively mismatched couple was Cordell and Rachel Pixler.

The Pixlers were regulars at the Rexford. They had a table every Saturday night but frequently patronized the restaurant at other times as well. Cordell and Rachel usually brought other distinguished couples with them, including an occasional single, rotating the invitations among a close-knit group of friends and upper crust clients. Several bottles of fine wine, beginning with Cordell's favorite 2003 Belle Glos Pinot Noir were pulled from the Rexford's climate-controlled cellar on each occasion that the couple and their friends partied. And the party that evening seemed to be rolling right along, and hard, the tab mounting as pure business expense.

In contrast, the mood at the Foxworth-Lisenbe table was much more intimate and not nearly as costly. Two glasses of a medium-priced chardonnay were sipped, one each, along with a weighty gourmet burger and steak fries for me and blackened redfish for her. Glasses of free tap water finished the beverages for our meal. Despite my suspicion that he did not expect an overly generous tip, our waiter kept the bread tray filled with a variety of thick slices of sourdough, olive, and wheat nut varieties, most of which I consumed after dipping in Italian oil, also complimentary. I was happy to see the bread pudding recipe, the red-velvet mousse concoction, still listed on the menu; it had been one of my father's favorites. Kaylee and I split a healthy serving although I devoured more than my fifty percent. That night she had followed my conservative lead on the menu selections, but I never got any vibes that she considered me to be cheap. Girls don't like to eat and drink that much anyway.

Once the romantic meal inside the Rexford was over, the valet brought around my new Mustang. Probably somewhere toward the end of my burger, he had partially toweled off the car, drying the exterior from the residue of the rain shower that had begun before dinner. When he was careful to point out his attention to detail, I rewarded the teenager with an extra buck. In the well-lit entrance area, it was clear that there were few beads of water left to mar my shiny car, the replacement for the used Jag cremated at the steps of the Architzel estate.

So far, I felt that the evening had gone well with Kaylee. The time was only shy of nine o'clock, certainly too early to go in. The streets of Larkspur were quiet as we drove nonchalantly in no direction in particular. Honestly, even though it was not a Jag, I was enjoying my Mustang, with or without Kaylee in it. The music system was top-notch, producing a full and resonant sound even with the top lowered, the temperature mild and breezy in the aftermath of a cool but heavy rain. Indeed, the inclement weather on the way to the restaurant had been a concern. However, the downpour did not spoil the ambience but served only to rinse away any exterior dust from my magnificent red vehicle.

The remaining beads of rain gleamed like prisms that night from the hood as my new wheels glittered under the bright streetlights of Andrews Boulevard, one of the main thoroughfares of that section of Larkspur. Even Kaylee remarked that the way had been recently so well-lit by the Larkspur City Council that one almost did not need headlights to drive there at night. The mayor of Larkspur and his cohorts were proud of such recent efforts to deter crime and planned to keep those statistics low.

Exponential growth of any community is easily measured by its road expansion, and Larkspur at the time served as a prime example. That night, Andrews Boulevard was similar to many other passageways in the town and on its outskirts. Strewn along the boulevard were striped orange barriers, identifying the uneven road elevations between the expanded asphalt and revised lane markings. I remember my concern over maintaining the speed limit, not a burdensome chore considering the relaxed but anticipatory mood of the open-air drive.

Shortly after weaving into the next driving lane to miss one of the orange markers of an asphalt drop off, we approached the latest strip shopping center, which boasted a frozen yogurt and ice cream shop nestled between a Home Depot and a Target. Both Kaylee and I shared thoughts about more dessert as I signaled left and moved into the turn lane, heading for the bright neon lights of commercialism.

It seemed that most of Larkspur had a similar idea. Traffic was thick as vehicles of every description wandered in semi-organized order through the parking area of the shopping center as if it were a maze. Flashing blue lights abruptly interrupted this throng of evening shoppers trying to beat the ten o'clock closing, not a problem unless those lights were flashing at you.

My knee-jerk reaction was to flee as Kaylee and I were draped in waves of revolving blue color, but I immediately thought better of it. A self-perceived law-abiding citizen, I instead pulled out of traffic into the nearest vacant parking space on the edge of what was actually the Home Depot section of the shopping center. I then stared over at Kaylee, whose eyes seem to share my bewilderment.

"Have you got one of those cards from your car insurance company? You know, proof of insurance?" she asked trying to hide her nervousness.

Actually the recently enacted and enforced Mississippi law requiring proof of automobile insurance had already caused a sudden sinking feeling in my chest. Was there such a document in that packet presented to me by the insurance agent? Arranged neatly in a shiny leather-like case, the collection of cards and papers was handed to me just after the newspaper photographers had captured the moment for posterity – a local hero receiving his unexpected but deserving reward for saving a dog. With much less fanfare, I had tossed the case into the glove compartment without checking the contents, assuming that my agent had put together whatever I would need. Reaching across Kaylee's waist to the door of the glove compartment, my fear was that the insurance guy's desire for publicity over the car key presentation had not extended to supplying me with the proper papers. Opening the door to the compartment, I was certain that this local hero, the one who tried in vain to save the old lady but instead rescued her yelping dog, would soon be slapped with a costly, non-negotiable traffic fine.

My concern was ill-placed.

"Sir, step out of the car." I had just grabbed the document packet, brushing across my date's smooth, slightly jittery, legs in the process.

"I was trying to get my proof-of-insurance card out for you," I explained to the small face in a blue uniform, peering inquisitively inside the car.

"You won't need that. Just get out of the vehicle, sir, and let me see your driver's license."

I glanced back over to Kaylee, who responded with an unhelpful shrug. Kaylee was as bewildered as I. There had been no speeding. I had made sure of it. Andrews Boulevard was a notorious speed trap, a fact learned on two prior but not recent personal experiences; pushing the limit now was made all the more impractical by the road construction.

The officer watched me closely as I exited the car, twisting her head slightly to talk indecipherably into a shoulder mounted radio. After retrieving my wallet from my back pocket, I handed her my license. She barely looked down at the smiling, laminated photograph before she asked, "Where have you been tonight?"

"Where have I been tonight?" I repeated with surprise. "Uh, my date and I have, uh, been out to dinner."

"So you've been drinking?"

"No, I haven't."

"But you just said that you'd been out to dinner."

"That's right. My date and I have been out to dinner."

The female officer smiled. "Then you have been drinking."

"What?" I asked more in a tone of shock than inquisition. Glancing back over to Kaylee, I added with control, "That doesn't necessarily mean that ... "

"If you have been to dinner then you have been drinking," the female officer declared as she muttered something else into her shoulder microphone.

Sipping one glass of wine slowly over a heavy restaurant meal was not my definition of drinking, so I stuck to my story, trying to respond unemotionally, in monotone. "Officer, I was not drinking," I repeated.

At the moment I was trapped before a dumpy, defiant policewoman in one of the busiest Saturday night sections of pavement in Larkspur: the parking lot of a popular, recently-opened shopping center. She seemed inexperienced and could not have been more than twenty-two or so, short, maybe five two, and definitely pushing the limit on any body weight regulations. Maybe police uniforms are meant to fit tight, no excess material to snag when chasing down criminals. From her austere demeanor, this protector of the people had assumed without a doubt that she had bagged one on the spot.

"Sir, you have been drinking." She sort of shifted her legs a bit, widening her stance and stiffening her thick, stubby legs as she continued. "I immediately detected the smell of alcohol when I approached your automobile. Besides, your eyes are bloodshot and your speech is slurred."

Up to that point of my legal driving career, I had experienced my share of close-call moving violations, predominately in the form of speeding tickets after one incomplete halt at a stop sign. Politely humbling myself with various excuses had barely, but successfully, seen me through most of those occasions as reasonable police officers generally let a nice guy like me go. However, this instance of being pulled over had caught me off guard. I was drowning, truly baffled over this current reason for having been stopped.

"My eyes are not bloodshot!" I shot back, somewhat surprised at my raised tone, certainly not my usual calm approach to such jammed situations.

"Sir, your eyes are very red, an obvious sign that you have consumed inebriating beverages."

"My eyes look red because they are inflamed. I'm being treated for a medical condition called *chemical conjunctivitis*," I countered. The policewoman (or should I say *police girl*?) kept staring at me as though in deep concentration although I never thought she actually absorbed anything I said. "I guess you don't read the newspaper, Officer. Anyway, I recently tried to rescue this elderly woman from a house fire and got blasted with thick smoke. As you might imagine, a lot of smoke hit my eyes and irritated them. Not good when you already wear contacts. My ophthalmologist has given me medication for the redness; it's just not working very well yet."

If the officer had been a follower of the local news, she was not going to let celebrity status interfere with her appointed duty. "Sir, you were demonstrating signs of intoxication by driving your vehicle recklessly."

Unsure if Kaylee remained close enough to hear all of the growing banter, particularly with all the moving parking lot traffic around us, I responded, "What do you mean *recklessly?*" My indignation was building as I fought to remain rational, or at least to appear that way. "My date and I were driving along the boulevard well within the speed limit." Kaylee noticed that I was gesturing toward her, magnifying her question over the length of the interaction with the officer. "Miss, there was no way to drive recklessly, especially with all the road construction and barriers set everywhere." Just as Kaylee reached for the handle to the front passenger door, another police cruiser pulled up against my Mustang, creating a parking space in an enthusiastic demonstration of inertia. He brushed so close to my new car, his blue lights draping the gleaming red paint, that I nearly screamed but thought better of it. Accordingly, an equally startled Kaylee was blocked from completely exiting the car and coming to my defense.

"Miss, stay in the vehicle please." With her right leg barely out of the partially opened side door, Kaylee immediately obeyed and retracted it.

"Do you want me to call someone, Sher?" Kaylee offered, yelling over the encircling and amplifying traffic noise. "I don't have my cell phone but if you'll give me yours ... "

Reflexively I reached deep into my right pocket, producing my stylishly thin, black flip phone, the replacement for the heavier cell that used to cradle in my poor Jag. The policewoman promptly confiscated it. "Hey! Wait a minute. I want to give that to my girlfriend so she can call a lawyer or someone."

Kaylee must have gathered the nerve to once again leave the car, this time lifting herself over the center console and scooting across the driver's seat. Promptly the officer in the other cruiser aborted this second attempt, reaching to place his hand on her shoulder. My date's fiery glare up at him made the contact brief.

"You'll get to make a call later," declared the woman before me that I was beginning to know from her badge as Officer Sleethe.

"Look, I don't understand this situation. I told you I have not been drinking. We have only been out to eat at the ... "

"We only had one glass of wine each!" A disgusted yell meant to be helpful came from Kaylee's direction as she lifted her body from the seat to project better. I rolled my eyes in response. *Damn girls, particularly honest ones.*

"That's what I thought," Officer Sleethe replied with satisfaction. "You **have** been consuming alcohol. And yep," she smirked, "no one ever has but one glass."

I looked in Kaylee's direction as she was placed back down into her seat once again by the helpful second officer.

Sleethe then continued, "Before I was interrupted, I was explaining that I have reason to believe that you have been driving under the influence."

"Well, I am not *under the influence*." By now, there was no way to camouflage my anger; no doubt my face and neck were as red as my smoke-irritated eyes. "And I was not driving recklessly!"

"Sir, you can take a field sobriety test here or come on down to the station for a breath analyzer level. If you fail the field test, then I'll give you the breath test to measure your level of intoxication."

Escalating to a wrenching nightmare, the whole situation there in the Home Depot parking lot resembled a bad dream. For some reason Kaylee had admitted the glass of wine each, totally blowing my abstinence argument in an attempt, I assumed, to alter my ineffective defense tactic against the driving drunk charge. However, maybe her reasoning was not way off base, I considered. After all, the restaurant's serving portion of chardonnay had been modest by any standard and had been consumed over a heavy meal, particularly for me. No way did I feel intoxicated, having a threshold of comparison from multiple previous experiences. Glaring down at this Officer Lyric Sleethe, I chose to stand my ground.

Suddenly the name on her badge seemed to stare angrily up at me from her uniform. Per protocol Sleethe had said her name at the moment she instructed me to get out of the car. But the identification was beginning to sink in. Officer Lyric Sleethe reeked of inexperience as well as defiance and was not about to let her catch go. I mentally replayed the frequently run television commercials sponsored by the Mississippi Highway Patrol – some big-chested, bruiser patrolman asking a scrawny male actor with tussled hair if he had been drinking, the actor with slurred speech playing inebriation for the Emmy while stumbling along an imaginary line, arms outstretched as though walking a circus tight rope.

"Okay. I'll take the test here." As I looked back at Kaylee for an ounce of moral support, she only could mouth, "I'm sorry, I don't know what to do," as she shrugged her soft, bare shoulders under the perceived admiration of the male officer hovering over her.

As 'sweet' Officer Sleethe rattled off memorized instructions to the field sobriety test, she explained that the other police officer would serve as the witness since the video equipment of neither cruiser was operational. This apparently was the cue for the second officer to move closer to the would-be ogre and me, leaving his patrol car as a tangential barrier to the convertible as though Kaylee, my accomplice, were going to hop over to the driver's position, start the engine of the sports car, and bolt without me.

While vehicles continued to encircle us in the parking lot, passengers and drivers alike gawking at the unenviable spectacle, I hoped that Kaylee would be attentive enough to be my witness. Considering my companion as an accomplice, Sleethe would no longer allow me audience with Kaylee as she remained nervously in the car. The people cruising around me were justifiably curious, drawn to the constantly flashing police lights of two cruisers and the shameless "drunk" fool getting what he deserved. As I did my best to keep my eyes from shaking horizontally during the nystagmus portion of the field sobriety test, I noticed several students gawking. A few even pointed at me.

The distraction caused by the uninvited audience only added to the embarrassment which worsened though the "tightrope" test. Later I would realize that I had misunderstood the directions, making that part of the quiz much more impossible than it had to be. Unfortunately, my overall failing grade was cinched with miscounting the number of steps required to walk the imaginary line. Because of that poor arithmetic, I practically stumbled into a pile of landscaping timbers, neatly stored inside a composite-plastic fence barrier within the parking lot. Even with that blunder, I mistakenly believed that my scholarly performance during the stand-on-one-leg test had redeemed the preceding, poorly executed physical feats. Tragically, my bonus score was likely squandered halfway through that segment when I almost started to giggle over what I considered the total absurdity of the situation: a dehumanizing spectacle for the hungry observer.

Overall I rated my performance well above that of the television commercial actors who on screen repetitively illustrated the perils of drinking and driving. Great was my relief that the horrendous ordeal of the test was successfully over and I had proven my sobriety. Tragically, Officer Sleethe did not concur with my self-assessment.

"Mr., uhhhh," she retrieved my driver's license from her shirt pocket and refreshed herself of my name, "Foxworth." To her, the name might as well have been Jones. After a confirming nod from her witness, 'Robo-cop' Sleethe continued in rote fashion. "After assessing your performance during the field sobriety test, I have confirmed that you are under the influence."

"You're joking. You've got to be." Once again I thought of Ashton Kutcher and my being punked. If only that could have been possible.

The short, squatty young girl in a police uniform directly in front of me did just that in response to my declaration.

"What's this all about? It's just crazy!" Frustrated and beginning to feel helpless, I started waving my arms around as though swatting flies all the while searching mentally for defensive arguments. "I am not under the influence. It's been raining, and ... and this asphalt is slippery. Besides, I don't wear these hard sole shoes often, and it's difficult to walk in them especially like this and in front of all of these people. That's the reason I didn't do well enough on your little tests to satisfy you." My friend Lyric still did not alter her facial expression from frozen. A frowning, elderly woman walking by the exposition filled in for the policewoman.

"Anyway, I'm supposed to get a phone call, get a chance to call a lawyer."

Officer Sleethe stepped back from me a bit as she motioned to the male officer who had served as witness to the proceedings. I studied him closely as he walked slowly toward me in response, not seeming to share his partner's pressing attitude. Dutifully producing the handcuffs, I could sense a bit of embarrassment in his demeanor — but not enough discomfiture to prevent his securely handcuffing me. While Kaylee was left sitting alone in the Mustang, I astonished myself by instinctively putting my hands in proper as he came to constrain me.

"You can take the breathalyzer test down at the station," she explained, "since you failed field sobriety."

"I didn't fail 'field sobriety,' " my repetitive inflection dangerously close to mockery. "These things are on my wrists too tight, really hurting my upper arms, almost pulling my shoulders out of socket," I complained while her accomplice escorted me to the awaiting backseat of Sleethe's cruiser.

"Handcuffs aren't meant to be comfortable," she retorted as the prisoner was pried into government-issue car with a gentle shove by the male officer, who also supplied a wry smile.

Straining to look back toward Kaylee, it was impossible at that point to see her face. I wanted to talk with her, just discuss the situation, put our heads together and try to figure out what to do next. Not sure if she had any money to hire a taxi or even to use for a pay phone to call for help, handcuffed Sher Foxworth was helpless as a gentleman. *What a shitty date. What a big loser I got mixed up with* ... That was what I assumed a lesser girl would have said about the state of her association with me. But somehow I knew Kaylee Lisenbe was different.

As expected, the backseat of the police car was stuffy, reeking of stale sweat, and seemed strangely familiar. My chauffeured ride was outfitted with the classic metal barrier between the front and backseats just like that seen on television crime dramas. My relentless complaints about the tight steel grips crushing my wrists went ignored, although I thought I heard her say something under her breath about adding shackles.

"Well, since you're going to paralyze my upper body, you might as well give me a little air back here." Silently, without even moving her head, Officer Sleethe threw me a bone and complied. The left rear passenger window lowered electronically, sufficiently enough to emit a stream of fresh air but not nearly enough to allow a man to squeeze out any part of his body.

By then I was exhausted. My head started to spin from all that had recently unfolded: the almost laughable telephone meeting with the fire marshal; a romantic, but fairly economical dinner with Kaylee in the shadow of the Pixlers; and the embarrassing aerobic stunt just performed for what must have been over half of the population of Larkspur. My thoughts were definitely clouded; maybe I truly was drunk.

From that point forward, I could no longer think logically about how to handle the police situation or clearly decipher what had just happened to me. My confusion as to why I had been pulled over by the lovely Lyric Sleethe was shortly answered. En route to police headquarters she pulled her cruiser and prisoner into a grocery store parking lot, still brightly illuminated although the store was already closed. Just under the sign advertising *BUD-LIGHT TWELVE PACKS $9.99 WITH SEPARATE TWENTY-FIVE DOLLAR PURCHASE*, another lone police cruiser sat waiting in an otherwise empty space.

A tall, brawny, male dude exited the vehicle and walked to my side of Lyric's squad car. Up to that point, I had not been afraid – instead, predominately aggravated – no, more than aggravated – pissed-off. Lyric sprang from her commandant post in the driver's seat to greet the muscular policeman dressed in another example of tight-fitting police attire. Anxiously, I peered out the window across busy Andrews Boulevard, watching the cars fly by – driven by law-abiding citizens oblivious to the peril of the criminal chained in the squad car under the beer-for-sale sign. Maybe a few of them noticed the anonymous silhouette confined to the backseat but certainly had no concern at all about the unknown wrongdoer. No doubt they were all relieved that the streets of Larkspur were now safer, cleared of another scumball, and happy that they themselves were not in the rear of that squad car. The two officers, who seemed to be devoting all of their taxpayers' salary to my debacle, were in no way concerned with the other passers-by. Several vehicles were obviously speeding, so much so that if tonight's navigation of my automobile had been an example of reckless driving, the entire town might as well have been locked up with me.

Lyric got out of the car and strutted in a roundabout way to where I was pinned in her backseat. Bending slightly to peer through the window into my domain, she stretched the stitching of her dark polyester uniform as her jellied abdomen and thighs pressed against the side of the squad car. "Mr. Foxworth," she addressed me while referring to her ticket pad, "Captain Diablo will be talking to you in just a minute. He was on-duty downtown and first observed you driving recklessly. He then radioed ahead to alert me."

Of course, I had noticed no police car downtown before or after we had patronized the restaurant at the Lexford. "Hey, look, Officer Sleethe, these handcuffs, they're really killing me. Making my hands swell." This time, Sleethe did not even bother to respond to the whining – verbally, that is.

The muscle-bound cop approached me, not looking up from the pad of paper tickets he was holding. "Mr. Foxworth, I followed you from downtown." He scribbled in. "You did not have your car lights on."

"Didn't have my lights on? That's nuts ... I mean ... There's no way that could be right, uh, sir. I believe I would have known if my lights were off." The brain synapses were firing indiscriminately, my mind racing, searching. Lights were off? No way.

"Sir, we are charging you with driving without proper illumination." Diablo corroborated in a sideways glance over to his female accomplice, his hesitation too slight for someone inebriated to catch. "Yes, that's right. That's the reason your vehicle was stopped."

I wished again for Kaylee; I wanted to discuss the whole mess with her. There was no one to help me argue with those people, to help me make sense of what they were saying. The car lights – the instrument panel had seemed dim as we drove from the Rexford toward the ice cream parlor, but I had not thought much of it at the time. Sweating and aching in the back seat of Sleethe's cruiser, I mentally surmised that because Andrews Boulevard was so well illuminated that the main headlights of my new Mustang could have been off or at least only dimmed and I might not have noticed. Thank you, city council for improving Larkspur, I thought to myself.

But if the headlights had been off in the first place, how did that happen? I remembered from my abbreviated new owner's orientation that when set properly the headlights illuminate automatically in the dark, a feature not available on my older, more familiar, but now incinerated Jaguar. During the early evening rain shower, I had activated the windshield wipers of the modern Mustang but did not recall adjusting the headlight controls positioned on the opposite side of the steering column. However, I was certain that I had not knowingly changed any of the dashboard settings except to adjust the windshield wiper speed. Maybe the restaurant valet had fooled with the headlight controls, even inadvertently, I guessed.

"Captain, sir. This other officer told me that I had been stopped because I was driving recklessly. But there's no way I was."

Captain Diablo darted his eyes toward his female underling. A cast of inquisitive exasperation or maybe even irritation was obvious to the callous, hardened criminal handcuffed in the backseat, handcuffed so tightly that his brain's cognitive reasoning was not receiving blood circulation fast enough to think through the predicament.

"Oh, yes, that's correct. You were driving ... recklessly." The captain reared his torso erect to bolster his support for the other officer's assertions as his eyes darted quickly back and forth toward her, his words a repetition of Officer Sleethe's information. Otherwise his facial features remained hard, defiant, and purposeful as I looked at him in disbelief. "In fact, I will testify in court to that fact. You were driving recklessly," he summarized while offering a subtle nod to his accomplice in what I considered a trumped-up charade. The travesty was documented with the long, rectangular slip of thin paper he tore from his ticket pad and started to hand over to me through the now fully lowered cruiser window. Before I could reach for it with my mouth to illustrate that my upper extremities were approaching paralysis, he thought twice and said, "Officer Sleethe will give you a copy of this later with your other papers."

Starting to retreat to the sanctuary of his own police cruiser, Diablo leaned forward toward my backseat cell and gave me a visual once over, although he seemed to be sniffing the air around me as much as visually inspecting his prey. I was relieved to see him leave as he sped away under an important blanket of flashing blue lights. Officer Lyric Sleethe resumed the commandant's position in the front seat, then pulled her vehicle back onto

Andrews Boulevard in a manner much less dramatic than that from the Home Depot.

Crammed physically and crushed emotionally in my seat directly behind my female captor, I longed again for an advisor: someone to make some decisions for me. Kaylee had been no help; she couldn't have been. I'll never know if she made things worse by admitting that each of us had a glass of wine. The predicament was overwhelming: stopped for unknowingly driving without my headlights on, accused of driving under the influence, supposedly failing a field sobriety test that I thought almost a joke, now handcuffed although I could no longer feel my wrists to be sure. Not only had this local hero been humiliated amidst a swarm of worshippers out for an evening of Target and Home Depot shopping, but being branded with a DUI conviction would do wonders for any future reapplication to medical school.

Lyric Sleethe pulled us under a backdoor canopy to the Venice County Detention Center, a structure sporting a speckled stone exterior that I had passed on other more pleasant occasions. Each time I had snubbed it as an endpoint for the lowest of the low, the scourge of society – home to the deadbeats of citizenry, certainly no one you knew or would ever want to know. As she opened the car door for me, I again mentioned how uncomfortable the handcuffs were. Completely ignoring me, she led me inside the building to a sort of check-in area.

"Hey, Lyric."

"Hi, Guys." Officer Lyric Sleethe was at home there, speaking to and laughing with all of her cohorts. She was particularly chummy with a prisoner outfitted in an orange jumpsuit who apparently was a trustee allowed to walk freely in the area. "I'll go out now and get ya'll your Smoothies," she called over to the four occupied cells filled with the types I expected to see in a place like this. There was no question that I was just another piece of white trash, another booking, another successful arrest and hoped-for DUI conviction to add to Lyric's march toward career advancement.

The obese gentleman sitting behind the check-in counter looked up at me suspiciously as Lyric handed him the paperwork documenting my crime against humanity. She left me to the whaleish attendant who commanded a rolling desk chair and strolled over to the guy in the orange jumpsuit. Their apparent thrill in seeing each other was so great that they nearly hugged. He's probably her brother, or better yet, boyfriend, I decided in disgust.

After studying the physical part of me he could see without lifting himself from his chair, the detention center clerk seemed to be forming his own mental assessment of my degree of inebriation. As he focused on making checkmarks in some diminutive, black boxes on yet another form, I noticed the unused telephone positioned just to my right. "I know my rights. I'm entitled to a telephone call," I pushed, although the demand sounded feeble, produced by a broken man.

Perturbed by the disturbance, the portly fellow glanced away from the papers and looked back up at me from his chair. "You'll get to make a call later, after we book you," he announced sarcastically.

"The officer wouldn't let me call an attorney earlier during this sham, sir. If you can believe what you see on TV, I think I am supposed to get to ... "

Blowing me off in interruption, he yelled over to another public servant sitting to his right, touting a terse complaint about a comrade coming in late again for work. As though I had not even spoken, he proceeded with the routine. "Empty your pockets including your wallet and take off your shoes," he directed to the newest, nameless prisoner placed before him on the other side of his counter.

"How am I supposed to empty my pockets while handcuffed?" I bantered. After Sleethe had confiscated my phone earlier during the ordeal, my only personal effects other than clothes were the wallet in my right back pocket and a few coins in the front right – the keys to my reward for being the town hero were, I hoped, still safe in the Mustang's ignition and under Kaylee's watchful eye.

The orange jumpsuit responded to the whale's motions and clumsily removed the wallet and coin change from my pockets. His lack of finesse in doing so had probably earned his admission to the joint. My renewed disappointment at not being freed from the cuffs to handle that maneuver myself had to be obvious even to the impersonal jail crew.

"When are they going to bring my friend back?"

"You mean your husband?" clarified the second officer who had witnessed for Sleethe and then been assigned to wait with Kaylee in the still busy parking lot where the stores have extended Saturday hours.

"Oh, he's not my husband," Kaylee corrected. "But I do need to go and check on him."

"After he's booked they'll let him make a phone call. Maybe he'll call you then."

"Well, he does have a cell phone, but I left mine in another purse so there's no way he can call me."

"Then it won't be a problem will it because Officer Sleethe confiscated his cell phone."

"Confiscated his cell phone? You're kidding!"

"That's procedure, ma'am," he explained to the youthful woman who had since been allowed to exit the Mustang and was now leaning lightly against it. She was appealing, nice-sized breasts, tight butt, giving him the impression of a party girl. "Also we're going to have to get that car of yours removed. The Department can't be responsible for it. We can't just abandon it here in a private commercial lot. Besides, it's parked illegally."

"Illegally?"

"Yeah, look." The officer pointed toward the Mustang and its left front and back tires, positioned just over the white stripe defining a designated slot.

"Oh, since Sher left his keys in the ignition, I can fix that little problem for you, officer. Anyway, I need to drive down to the police station and pick him up. Surely by now they must be finished with that breath test." Leaving the policeman, she moved to the driver's side door and announced while opening it, "Sher had to have passed. What a nightmare this whole thing has been for him and me! I'll be so glad when it's over so ... "

"You can't drive that car, Ma'am," he interrupted.

"What? Why not?" Kaylee said almost indignantly as she stepped partially into the vehicle.

"Because you've been drinking alcohol tonight. You admitted it."

"Drinking alcohol? I said I had had one glass of wine. That's not enough to ... "

"Yes, ma'am. That's right. Yeah, we know. Supposedly your friend consumed one glass of wine, too, and, well, just look what has happened to him. Arrested and carried off in a police car. I'm sorry but this vehicle here will have to be towed."

Fumbling with my wallet and loose change, the guy behind the counter, who appeared to be growing fatter by the minute, counted the few greenbacks formerly in my possession. After filling out yet another paper form and affixing it to a long brown envelope, he inserted the modest amount of money and licked the envelope closed. He scribbled my name across the middle of the package with a black felt tip pen and then stored the treasure in plain view on the top of a low table behind him. As I observed this ritual, the handcuffs felt even tighter as my wrists along with my indignation continued to swell against the strangling metal.

"Come on over here to the breathalyzer room," she directed. Officer Sleethe had returned, delivering variously flavored Smoothies to the outstretched arms of the confined regulars. The concoctions were expected treats, all for good behavior and at taxpayer expense. She marched me down an adjacent hall where a diminutive room waited, complete with a narrow, barred window embedded in the upper area of its door. The cramped space housed a leased alcohol sensor, calibrated daily and frequently updated by the manufacturer. At the last minute, my request to keep my shoes on was granted, preventing a forced, stocking-foot walk across the length of the filthy precinct building toward the analyzer room. This charitable gesture, I was informed, was granted against policy for jailhouse arrestees.

"Thanks for tossing a crumb to lowly little ol' me," I snidely wanted to say to Lyric and her gang but restrained myself. Nonetheless, as we entered the small space for the breathalyzer test, I resumed the arguments against my incarceration. "Look, I am not drunk."

"Sir," she answered with rolling eyes, "we are not talking about *drunk*. We're talking about being under-the-influence."

"This is all a big mistake," I interrupted. "I'm not under-the-influence now, and never have been during this whole mess." I wanted to add a few expletives to my countering, but again resisted.

"There was enough evidence at the scene, sir, to show that you broke the law by operating a vehicle while impaired. Also you were driving recklessly," Sleethe spoke slowly during the summarization, as succinctly as her high school education would allow and as though I were in kindergarten.

"But I wasn't reckless. My automobile lights were on; it's just that I must have been driving using only the parking lights. I guess that somehow the automatic on/off sensor controls got screwed up during the day." Pushing on with my theory developed on the ride to the detention center, I detected no sign of her believing my explanation. However, I felt I had nothing to lose by trying. "If I was driving without the car lights turned on, it was not intentional. Since the boulevard was so well lit by streetlights, I guess my date and I didn't notice. Besides, I haven't had my car all that long, so I'm not that familiar with the dashboard controls."

Lyric cut me off before I could offer more excuses and elaborate on how a town hero could never have committed such acts. However, I chose not to push further along those lines, growing to realize that her kind assumed such honorable things to be banalities. I would later learn that she and the other members of her department craved catching big fish (state congressmen, judges, displaced law enforcement officers – individuals much more significant than I) – so even if she had followed my saga in the news she would not have given a flip.

"Beginning with when I pulled your vehicle over, this form lists tonight's information documented about your behavior and appearance." Lyric Sleethe pointed to a pad of paper bound in triplicate that she had slapped on the small table near an awaiting chair.

I looked down at the yellow piece of paper on top, decorated with handwritten check marks preceding items on a long list. The first item drew my immediate attention: *Eyes Bloodshot.*

"Hey, I explained to you why my eyes are red. I've been seeing an ophthalmologist for conjunctivitis; that disease makes your eyes red. I'm taking some prescription medication for it."

Sleethe grinned *Gotcha.* "You've already admitted to consuming a glass of wine. Well, I ran some history on you. You're a science teacher at the private school. I myself didn't go there, parents couldn't afford it; I graduated from public school. Anyway, someone as smart as you especially should know not to drink alcohol if you're taking prescription medicine."

"But the medication is eye drops. Eye drops! Besides, I haven't admitted to any alcohol. My date did."

Kaylee decided not to argue any further with her policeman babysitter. The guy seemed nice, more personable than the short bitch squeezed into the uniform a couple of sizes too snug. During their awkward parking lot conversation, he divulged his own lack of certification in administering the sobriety exam and through an apologetic demeanor suggested that his precinct associate had been overly zealous in the DUI arrest.

Suddenly Kaylee thought about her father, the marshal of the Larkspur Fire Department, and her mind refocused on solving the unfair dilemma. She shared my horror over being on public display and at the mercy of the police, particularly when one glass of wine had not affected our demeanors. As a city official, her father should have connections, maybe connections reaching to the police department.

She had to do something.

"Officer, are you going to arrest me, too?" she asked as the young policeman started to light a cigarette.

"No, ma'am. You haven't broken any laws that I know of."

"Am I free to go then?"

"Well, yes, ma'am, you are. You just can't drive that car, any car right now because you've been drinking ... "

"Wait a minute," she interrupted with her right arm extended toward him as though to stop traffic. "We're not going over all that again. I've enjoyed our little chat, but this is going nowhere." Turning around for her cell phone believed left in my car, she remembered aloud, "Damn, I changed purses right before Sher picked me up, and my cell phone is in my other purse."

Determined to get help, Kaylee started across the parking lot toward Target and Home Depot, leaving the young policeman to admire her tight gait from the rear. "Do they still have payphones in stores?" she asked to no one in particular as she scurried away, hoping that tonight's purse at least contained change for the phone.

"The mandatory twenty minute waiting period since booking you is over. I can administer the breath analyzer test to you now." During those twenty minutes that seemed like twenty hours, I had been sitting in a small chair in a poorly ventilated room across from Officer Lyric Sleethe, staring at the name badge resting just inside a red and white monogram: *LARKSPUR, THE FRIENDLY HOMETOWN*.

"Why do you need to do this breath test on me anyway? You're already sure that I'm drunk. What is the real story here? Do you need to register a monthly minimum number of these tests as positive or at least put a certain number of citizens through this ordeal to earn a higher police rank?" My attitude and demeanor had deteriorated from organized debate to purely cynical.

Sleethe ignored me in well-practiced, professional fashion (however, I imagined a suppressed smirk) as she removed a plastic tubular device from an adjacent cabinet. My wrists and forearms had been confined long enough by the handcuffs that I could no longer feel the restriction. "As you can see, this blower is sealed and numbered, ready for the next test subject. And that would be you, Mister ... " (again she had to refer to the information recorded on the top sheet of her Uniform Traffic Ticket pad) " ... Foxworth. Once that timer there goes off, you have to inform me of your decision about the breath analyzer. That is, whether or not you're going to take it. If you refuse, it's an automatic ninety-day driver's license suspension."

"What happens if I take that breathing test and pass?"

"Then you might be released. But ... "

"But, what?"

"Based on the evidence I have collected so far: failed field sobriety test, bloodshot eyes, slurred speech, smell of alcohol, belligerent attitude, I have enough evidence to book you for *Driving Under the Influence*, even without an alcohol level above 0.08." She seemed to savor each point as she ran down her recorded list, touching each item proudly with the pen tip.

Judging from Officer Sleethe's autocratic manner, I believed that she would follow through with that plan.

And she did.

Kaylee arrived at the detention center shortly after my fingerprinting. Remembering a male movie actor's well-publicized mug shot leaked after his DUI arrest, I had tried to straighten my hair the best I could without a comb and mirror. Smiling for my own arrest photograph earned a chortle from the morbidly obese man who worked behind the reception counter and who also doubled as the precinct's photographer. By that time Police Officer Lyric Sleethe had finished with me and disappeared, no doubt returning to the crime-ridden streets of Larkspur to round up other criminals out for quiet dinners with their girlfriends.

Fortunately, I did not have to join the long-term, incarcerated residents housed down another hall. Thirteen hundred and sixty dollars of bond money secured my release.

Fire Marshal Lisenbe got his money back when the charges against me were dismissed by the presiding judge, touting a technicality surrounding my arrest and processing that I never understood or questioned. Likewise, my mug shot and fingerprint records disappeared along with Officer Sleethe's completed forms. As it turned out, not only did the marshal play a lot of golf, but he had card buddies, too. One of those close buddies was that circuit judge assigned to my DUI case, a judge who also doubled as a heavyweight over the police department.

To supplement the news that my life of crime had been erased, Fire Marshal Lisenbe also brought a contract by my apartment, enlisting me as the newest member of his department, contingent of course on successful completion of the fire academy down in Storck.

Chapter
9

•••

THE SCRAPBOOK

My grandfather was at home that afternoon in his den, hovering above a shipping carton and holding a box cutter.

"I guess you heard that I got a job." In his somewhat muted response there was not even a hint at the circumstances leading up to my trading a DUI charge for a stint as a fireman.

"Yeah, Tom Lisenbe was at the Nineteenth Hole today. I guess he thinks he's got a future son-in-law on the hook, too."

"My crash course at the Fire Academy starts in a couple of weeks. The marshal says I shouldn't have any problem with the physical or mental training aspects." Looking down at the cardboard crate, I inquired, "Can I give you a hand with that?"

"I ordered one of those DVD players from Great Buy. I had all the old family super 8 movies converted to DVD, all the ones with your grandmother and with your dad when he was little. Cost me a bundle. The early home movies were silent, if you can believe that. Later I bought a film camera that had sound. Of course, all of that was before those camcorders came around."

He pointed over to a package sitting on a nearby table that contained the Foxworth family DVDs, then reached down with the knife and slit open the box, exposing the player's white Styrofoam packaging. "You wanna help me with this? Putting electronic stuff together has never been my forte. I just like to use it."

Within thirty minutes we had the DVD player hooked up to the den TV. It had been years since my grandfather had looked at any of the home movies, and I certainly had never seen any of them. Despite the fact that the quality of the faded super 8 film was considered state-of-art for the late sixties and early seventies, its age was accentuated by the video conversion.

I watched a part of the video with my grandfather: my father's eighth grade and high school graduations, some of his junior high basketball games, my parents' wedding reception. The most poignant, at least for my grandfather, was that of the medical school commencement exercises, held outdoors that year at Harvard. Even with the faded color intensity extracted from that thin, brittle movie film, one could still appreciate the blooming spring trees bursting in glorious backdrop for my father's valedictory address. Since there was no audio, one could only imagine the truths, hopeful inspiration, and gratitude that Sheridan Smith Foxworth, Jr., MD, was articulating.

Despite the jumpy-frame technique characteristic of those Foxworth documentaries, my grandfather displayed some hope of more talented home movie production by including a close-up of my still sane grandmother. Sitting proudly in the audience during Dad's speech, she was basking in celebrated honor over her only child's achievements, her infinite motherly pride obvious in the facial expressions originally captured within reels of deteriorating film.

As the DVD played on to other jerky scenes of parties and holidays, Granddad stood morosely from his chair, placed a small file folder on the coffee table, and walked toward the kitchen. Quietly, almost to himself, he said something about getting a beer from the refrigerator. One was not offered to me, but by then I sensed he felt all alone in the room. The file which he had apparently been reading before I arrived to catch the DVD presentation fell open when it settled on the table, carelessly exposing the contents before me. Several yellowed, double-spaced typed pages lay there. The paper seemed moist in a few areas and the print smeared in spots of diameter just large enough to be covered by a spreading teardrop. Before I picked up the first page to read it, I looked toward the kitchen pathway to check if Granddad was returning. There was no sign of him.

The pages were a typed manuscript of that Harvard speech, probably the original from which my father had read in the video. It was indeed well written, allowing me to place words with the silent presentation still playing in my head. The address predicted success for the Harvard graduates as long as they applied themselves. Dad detailed that no one sitting in those chairs below him or on stage with him lacked the ability to succeed and that the world would expect much from them. The one thing he failed to speak to was fate and how chance, followed by just plain bad luck, can screw things up.

Surprising myself, I began to cry just as my grandfather had been doing, my own tears falling onto the yellowed pages, mingling with his.

Many years after that graduation, Mrs. Ridley delighted in seeing the Harvard medical school diploma on Dad's office wall. This was the doctor who would grant her daughter the beauty that surely God had meant for her. After meeting with Dr. Dan Foxworth for the initial consultation, she had delighted over the choices available in improving her daughter's appearance: more prominent chin, ears pinned back, nose bobbed, breasts enhanced and lifted, thighs liposuctioned, sagging upper arms corrected with a procedure called *brachioplasty with skin excision* – not to mention a tummy tuck. Developing an obsession of near perfection for poor Flowers Ridley, her mother cut pictures of attractive body parts from fashion and gossip magazines, mounting them on poster board attached to a smiling head shot of Flowers from a church retreat. Charity Ridley regretted that she could not extend her daughter's makeover to shortening of height, but then a lot of models were tall. Absolutely, Mrs. Ridley was certain of it. As a result of this wonderful doctor's skill, a New York modeling contract was possible, if not probable, for her daughter. No longer would Flowers' exemplary SAT and ACT scores be necessary for her to advance in life – no, not after the plastic surgeon fixed her.

Dr. Foxworth had infatuated Charity with his kindness and sincere manner toward her and Flowers. Even though digital computer imagery in plastic surgery practices was not so much in vogue then, the before and after patient images that Dad had provided reassured them as they scheduled the surgery. He explained that Flowers' procedures would be performed in an outpatient setting, inside his nearby comfortable, attractive, and state-of-the-art plastic surgical center.

As the assistant worked the camera Dr. Foxworth explained, "We're taking these before pictures, Flowers, because no one will recognize you after I'm through with your surgery, not even your mom." He chuckled and everyone in the room joined in.

The morning of the big day, Charity Ridley could not conceal her excitement over her intelligent but drab daughter's upcoming beauty. While she herself had not slept the night before, tossing and turning, Flowers snored right up to the 4 a.m. alarm. As promised, the limousine was waiting out front to whisk them away to a prompt 5:30 arrival at the Foxworth Center for Cosmetic and Surgical Body Enhancement. The pre-admissions nurse had been specific in her instructions: the surgery schedule was run efficiently throughout the day, and being on time was of paramount importance.

Gone that morning was the Pierce Brosnan look-alike. Instead, a well-worn nurse, an army-sergeant type, greeted them at the pre-operative check-in department. Her demeanor was more cordial than suggested by her appearance, allowing Charity to warm up to her after a few minutes of the nursing assessment review. Conversely, Flowers continued her rather aloof attitude to the whole process, a disposition more typical of a teenager than someone who was to undergo surgery.

"Good morning, Ridleys," my father greeted Flowers and her mother in the private pre-op room once the patient had undressed and changed into the surgical gown provided by the sergeant. She felt secure under the thin, but fresh smelling, sheet covering the patient bed. There were a dozen fresh, though out-of-season, pink roses on the bedstand near the door and colorful original artwork arranged on the wall. The attention to decorative detail and the homey, personal touches to the place continued to mystify and impress Charity Ridley. The entire ambience, even the somewhat controlling nurse that morning, reinforced her belief that her only child was in good hands and was soon to be transformed into a gorgeous woman.

"Now, what we're going to need you to do is please remove your surgical gown and then stand up beside your bed unclothed so …"

"Why?" Flowers interrupted my father before her mother had the opportunity.

Forcing practiced patience, my father answered, "So that we can make a few marks on your skin to use as a guideline during your procedures. We want everything to be just right so that you'll heal perfectly when we finish." Flowers cast her eyes down in embarrassment while the doctor drew all over her body with a black surgical marker. As the felt tip pen tickled her breasts and the nipples hardened, she experienced an element of pleasure foreign to her. The lines sketched near her pubic area and down along the inside and outside of her thighs produced such twinges that Flowers jumped as she stood before him, crossing her legs in reflex. "Try to be still, I'll be through in a minute," the plastic surgeon calmly added with intense concentration, not even glancing at the girl's already diagrammed face as he spoke.

"Oh, he's wonderful, a master," Charity Ridley muttered quietly.

"Flowers, next we'll need to get you to turn around so that I can see your buttocks area."

"Why?" Both mother and daughter said in unison.

"'Cause we need to finish marking your buttocks area for the liposuction and lift we're going to do there."

"But, Doctor, I didn't know you were going to do that, too!" Mrs. Ridley interjected with excitement even though she was privately concerned over any additional cost. The package of procedures she had negotiated with the business manager of the plastics center had already nearly depleted her retirement fund; there would not be enough money left to pay Dr. Foxworth for anything more than had previously been planned or discussed.

"When I was reassessing the file last evening, I realized that to get the overall result that you want, that Flowers wants, we need to do this work to her posterior as well." Dr. Dan Foxworth had been in practice long enough that he could practically read clients' minds. "Please don't be concerned about any additional cost. The work to the buttocks area won't take long. We'll simply include it as part of your total quote."

Dad noticed that the mother seemed relieved and had resumed breathing. "Also we may want to do a little work to the adipose tissue under the chin," he continued. "Right here in the front of the neck. Regarding the expense – same goes for that, too."

Relieved, Charity nodded while Flowers grimaced and rolled over to expose her flabby derrière. She laughed aloud during the crafting of thick black circles on her rear.

For hours Charity Ridley waited for daughter Flowers to emerge from surgery: through the continental breakfast served gratis in the guest lounge, the brunch-time drinks and snacks (some woman in a white apron even offered her a Bloody Mary, which she declined), and the suggestion of Creole shrimp or chicken Caesar salad for lunch. As each hour dragged, Charity ate her fill of the complimentary food, more to calm her growing uneasiness than from hunger. The procedures were taking much longer than expected, or at least longer than she had expected. A voice through an intercom speaker provided periodic updates: "Everything is going great!" or "Your daughter is doing just fine," or "Sweetie, we'll call you back soon with another update," or "Dr. Dan is moving right along. Won't be much longer at all." By the time Flowers was finally admitted to the post-surgical recovery room, her mother had finished off three glasses of wine offered later by the lady in the white apron and had started a fourth.

The wine buzz dulled the motherly shock of seeing Flowers encased from top to bottom and front to back in compression garments, including bra, girdle, and layers of tight elastic bandages. What appeared to be some type of sling was curiously encircling her daughter's neck and running up the sides of her face, covering both cheeks. Charity was not surprised to find the IV bag containing clear fluids and hanging on a pole mounted at the top of the bed. However, the chardonnay haze vanished as her eyes were drawn to the smaller bag suspended adjacent to the intravenous solution. Marked *PACKED RED BLOOD CELLS UNIT 3* the container was nearly empty, its upper portion stained dark maroon.

As Charity regained consciousness on a stretcher next to

her daughter, the recovery room nurse explained that she had collapsed at the foot of her daughter's bed, for whatever reason the staff was unsure. Dr. Foxworth had instructed the nurses to monitor the mother's vital signs, just as they were doing for Flowers, all readings of which had remained stable.

Informed by the recovery nurse that the girl's mother was alert, Dad promptly came to the room. He explained to Mrs. Ridley that after she collapsed he had detected no obvious problems during a brief physical exam of her.

"Sweetie, we believe you had a syncopal episode; you just plain ol' passed out," the recovery nurse clarified in a comforting tone.

"Flowers ... how is my Flowers?"

"Your baby is fine. She's waking up some, just like you are!" This time the recovery room nurse laughed in a silly octave. "I think you saw those bandages and got all excited for no reason. No reason, at all!"

"It's just that I saw this bag, this bag of blood hanging there on the IV pole. I didn't know anything about her getting blood," Charity interrupted weakly.

"Oh, that. Well, Dr. Foxworth got into some bleeding during the lipo of her buttocks and decided that your baby would heal better if she got a little blood transfusion. But don't worry, Sweetie, he got the bleeding stopped during the surgery. She'll be fine."

With a slightly more serious demeanor, the nurse stressed, "Because of your little spell this evening, Mrs. Ridley, the doctor wants you to get yourself checked real good and real soon by an internal medical specialist."

"But this surgery was supposed to be so simple, so easy on Flowers." Charity was feeling stronger now, although her head was beginning to pound. She sat up on the stretcher and stared over at her daughter. Flowers had been extubated since Charity had passed out, so the fact she was now breathing without a tube down her throat eased her mother somewhat.

"We're going to keep Flowers overnight in the guest quarters next door and keep her real comfortable. That way, we can keep an eye on her, and on you, too, for that matter!" The nurse giggled as she left to process the transfer paperwork, leaving alone the semiconscious patient and her dumbfounded mother.

The next morning the same jovial nurse brought a breakfast tray for the patient, who was still too sedated to know whether or not she was hungry. However, once the patient-controlled analgesia system was discontinued along with the IV fluids, Flowers began to perk up – but too late for the food. Charity had eaten the bacon and fried eggs while polishing off a whole pot of hot coffee, hoping to calm her hangover.

"Sweetie, we're gonna take some of these nasty ol' bandages off so that your doctor can take a little peek at his handiwork." The nurse unwrapped much of the younger Ridley's face as a gawking Charity fought back the tears, not sure if the emotions were of fear or anticipated joy. Ever since she had pursued the dream of achieving physical beauty for her simple daughter, Charity had assumed the result would be spectacular. After all, she had selected the best doctor and surgical facility available anywhere.

Despite the swelling and bruises, her precious child's manmade beauty was immediately obvious to the loving mother, overcoming her alcohol-withdrawal headache as well as the first impulse to swoon in encore as the bandages were discarded. Flowers' new face was not only an anticipated shock for Charity, but the nurse seemed flabbergasted as well.

"Oh, Dr. Foxworth has really outdone himself this time. Young lady, you're goin' to be gorgeous once you heal up." She giggled even louder. "That Nicole Kidman better watch her back once you get out there!"

"Ma'am, can I have a pain shot? My behind hurts really bad," Flowers managed to squeeze into the conversation.

The sympathetic nurse altered to a motherly tone, "Oh, for sure, Sweetie, that's from all that liposuction that Dr. Dan did on your buttocks area."

"Gosh, I didn't know he was going to do anything to me back there. Ahhh, please hurry with that shot, please. I can barely move. I'm in so much pain."

Charity Ridley was forced away from her daughter's agony as she sought relief in the view from the picture window across the room. Normally the landscape of blooming plants and other lush vegetation framed there would have appeared crisp and calming. However, through the tears of pain shared with her daughter, the detailed gardens appeared not at all inviting, but instead foggy and superfluous. Strangely, she no longer felt a wave of nausea over the aftermath of her daughter's operation and all that surrounded it. Instead, her queasiness in that recovery area was replaced by gnawing, growing guilt.

The remorse over her daughter's ordeal lessened as the two returned home with all medical and surgical bills paid-in-full. There had been no additional expense incurred from the longer time required in surgery or from the extra IVs or blood transfusion. Charity resumed her classroom teaching, leaving Flowers at home to convalesce while lazily studying models' pictures in fashion magazines. This time the daughter looked forward to looking just as fit and ravishing as the stars, once her healing was completed and all bandages permanently removed.

As is sometimes the case, the first episode went unnoticed. Deep in the valves of the lower left leg, some platelets within her own blood aggregated to form a nidus: a base for additional platelets to attach along with other blood particles to create a red fibrin thrombus. The body's thrombolytic system, generally protective in a healthy nineteen year old, worked diligently to dissolve the clot but was only partially successful. The incipient mass then incorporated itself into the wall of the vein, to wait.

The first symptoms of the initial episode were nonspecific: mild shortness of breath attributed to her urgent struggles for the toilet from too many Diet Cokes; chest pain during a deep breath, not surprising to Flowers since she hurt in so many other areas already; and a nagging cough thought due to her chronic sinus and allergy condition. She was still unconcerned even when she coughed up thick, pink sputum. During the time in between and during these events, Flowers took her pain pills, continued her deep breathing exercises as instructed by her doctor, and tried to remain self-sufficient.

Before long, minute pieces of the clot broke away from their origin deep in a left leg vein, and then raced through the circulatory system, searching to lodge in the most damaging, distant location. The target – the minute vessels in the outskirts of her lung tissue – was swiftly reached. A more dramatic chest pain was triggered, although Flowers was more alarmed by the blood-tinged sputum she suddenly choked up. The accompanying cough became repetitive as the teenager was strangled by shortness of breath.

A larger segment of blood clot promptly wedged into the lower lobes of the lung, completing the morbid process. The result was severe pulmonary compromise as her respiratory organs could no longer provide oxygen to the rest of the body's tissues. What followed was a functional failure of which even her nineteen-year-old heart could not overcome; the resistance to blood flow from the heart throughout the lungs had increased too greatly. As an end result, the body's tissues were smothered from the following hypoxemia as Flowers suffered overwhelming circulatory collapse due to lack of oxygen.

Charity Ridley found her precious daughter sprawled on the

kitchen floor in front of the opened refrigerator, the light still lit. Her right hand was stained with what appeared to be a small amount of thick blood and was against her chest. Flowers failed to respond to her mother's frantic screams which progressed to animal-like utterances.

Charity ran back through the living room and flung open the front door. "Somebody help us. Please! Dear God, will somebody please help us. It's my daughter!" As she grabbed the nearby cordless phone from the sofa table to call 911, a next-door neighbor gardening in his front yard heard the panicky screams. Throwing down his rake and bolting through the opened door, the man arrived in timely fashion to catch Charity Ridley immediately before she fell unconscious once again, this time to her own living room floor.

"What did you find?" my dad asked the pathologist as she joined the other physicians for lunch in the doctors' lounge. Usually Dad spent his entire day at his place, only venturing over to Larkspur Regional Hospital to answer an occasional consult or care for that rare post-operative patient whose surgery was not performed at the Foxworth Center for Cosmetic and Surgical Body Enhancement. However, today he made a point to join the ranks of the multispeciality physicians so that he could catch Dr. Grimes.

Helen Grimes, MD, based her pathology practice out of nearby Montclair, coming to Larkspur as needed when autopsies were ordered. Fortunately for the citizens of Larkspur, Dr. Grimes' services were not required on a fulltime basis. Per protocol, Dad and the social worker had encouraged Mrs. Ridley to consent to an autopsy regarding her daughter's unexpected and unexplained post-operative death. While at first she had seemed reluctant because of the additional medical cost, she abruptly changed her mind and signed the papers authorizing the procedure.

"PTE," the pathologist answered.

"Pulmonary thromboembolism?"

"Yes."

"But she's so young. I assumed that we'd find some sort of congenital heart defect or maybe that she had been abusing drugs or alcohol or something like that," Dad responded, appearing visibly shaken by Dr. Grimes' finding.

"There was peripheral occlusion of the pulmonary artery which resulted in parenchymal infarction in the lung. There was just no way for oxygenated blood to get out into the tissues of the lung. As a matter of fact that happens in about ten per cent of cases," Dr. Grimes clarified, taking another bite of her chicken salad sandwich on toasted wheat.

Trying to regain composure, Dad arose from the table where he was sitting alone with Dr. Grimes. He walked over to the beverage bar to dispense more iced tea, although he had no intention of consuming it.

"Death was sudden," the pathologist continued in unabated detail once he returned. "She never had a chance – although I suspect she may have had some smaller emboli in the days preceding which were not catastrophic, of course, and were probably only associated with minor, ignored symptoms."

"After being discharged from twenty-three hour observation, the girl never called my office with any physical complaints. As usual we saw her for dressing changes twice post-op, and she mentioned nothing out of the ordinary to my staff. I don't know what we could have done differently."

"I'm waiting for some more blood work to come back from the reference hematology lab. Maybe that will provide a clue," added Grimes.

The fragile human body possesses certain natural anticoagulants, molecules and proteins, which prevent circulating blood from clotting. Those untimely and sometimes morbid clots in the venous circulatory system can result from a deficiency in such blood thinning factors as protein C, protein S, and antithrombin III. The lack of these anticoagulants is responsible for ten percent of the venous thrombosis cases in young people, unfortunate instances where blood clots form unnecessarily and certainly unexpectedly – unexpectedly for both Flowers Ridley and her mother as well as for Dan Foxworth, MD – and unfortunate for different reasons.

Chapter
10
•••
THE COMPLAINT

Five business days after that informal doctor's lounge discussion between Drs. Grimes and Foxworth, it was delivered by certified mail. The office manager of my dad's plastic surgery practice signed for the austere document, the title of which read:

IN THE CIRCUIT COURT OF VENICE COUNTY, MISSISSIPPI

ESTATE OF FLOWERS NICOLE RIDLEY   *PLAINTIFF*

VS.   *CAUSE NO.: ND7911559-106*

SHERIDAN SMITH FOXWORTH, JR., MD, and
FOXWORTH CENTER FOR COMESTIC AND SURGICAL BODY ENHANCEMENT,
PLLC   *DEFENDANTS*

Jury Trial Demanded
COMPLAINT

The Complaint document was accompanied by an authorization form signed by Mrs. Charity Ridley. Her signature called for the Foxworth Center for Cosmetic and Surgical Body Enhancement to release an entire copy of the medical record of one Flowers Nicole Ridley. The recipient was to be the law firm of Cordell Pixler and Associates, LLC.

The practice manager waited until he was through with his morning patients before she broke the news to my father. The manager knew it was coming, as did my dad; they just did not know how soon. Once Flowers Ridley died, the manager had notified the medical liability insurance carrier of the adverse patient event, such reports being a requirement to maintain insurance coverage. But now that a plaintiff's attorney had made it official, the accusation of medical malpractice in the death of Flowers Ridley was in full force. What my dad and his practice manager had not yet considered was that a wrongful death suit against him was quickly to follow.

Throughout the later years of my student life at Larkspur Christian Academy, that patient contact with Flowers Ridley and the resulting aftershock had a profound effect on the Foxworth family. Every evening at home after school there was a pall over my house: no laughter, no pleasantries, barely any conversation between my father and mother, except for that necessary to raise their only child. The tension between them during the two years of medical malpractice legal proceedings was the cause of the unbearable, tortuous silence. They stopped socializing with most of their many friends. Messages left on the telephone answering machine for Dr. and Mrs. Foxworth or Dan and Kathleen went unanswered. Printed party and wedding invitations received in the mail were filed in the garbage can, most unopened.

Sometimes I would meander through the den, finding my dad sitting alone, lights dimmed, his face buried in his hands. Usually he would be muttering, "That poor girl." In the middle of those unrelated and rare conversations with my mother and me, as well as with his loyal friends and medical associates, his gaze would become distant, a characteristic unknown before the Ridley disaster. The guilt he suffered over the death of Flowers Ridley overwhelmed not only my father but also the rest of our tiny family – a guilt he bore despite the fact that the patient unknowingly carried a genetic tendency to form dangerous venous blood clots. Her body was a ticking bomb, harboring a medical complication that produced the massive pulmonary embolism resulting in her death – indeed a rarity, particularly for someone as young as Flowers Ridley.

As provided by his medical liability insurance carrier, a team of defense attorneys was hired on behalf of my father, their main objective being to cut the potential losses to the insurance company's balance sheet. Understanding this financial concern, Dad engaged a longtime friend to serve as his personal lawyer in overseeing the litigation process. Once the repeated legal depositions between the defense and plaintiff's attorneys ensued, the entire experience became even more draining for Sheridan Smith Foxworth, Jr., MD, and his family. Leading toward the medical malpractice trial, those depositions consumed hours upon hours, each minute spent dissecting the medical and surgical care rendered to Flowers Ridley, deceased. The pretrial investigative grilling unleashed by Cordell Pixler and his staff left deep scars on Dad's mental and physical well-being, or lack thereof.

Typically, Pixler brought a couple of assistants with him to each deposition: sometimes two men, sometimes two women, sometimes one of each, and usually of varying races. Each time the chief counsel was immaculately dressed, never repeating suits, silk ties, or French cuffed shirts. While the subordinates scribbled notes, Cordell always tossed the questions which began to run

together in macabre fashion, drafted to confuse and twist in
a probe to uncover damaging indecisiveness or careless
medical treatment.

Pixler pushed ahead relentlessly during the depositions as
though they were interrogations. "Why did the surgery last more
than eight hours, Doctor? ... What were you doing in there for
that long, in that cold, austere surgical suite, Doctor? ... Did you
advise Miss Ridley and her mother that the procedures would
drag into an all-day ordeal – well, did you, Doctor?... Tell me, sir,
when you operate in the buttocks region, how often do you let a
massive amount of human blood collect in the form of such a large
hematoma? ... Dr. Foxworth, you performed liposuction on Miss
Ridley's buttocks area and removed a good bit of her skin from
that spot. You plastic surgeons commonly refer to that as *a butt-
lift*, I believe. Please look through the patient's chart and show me
the consent for that procedure, Doctor."

The sad reality was that no separate written consent for that
surgical service existed since the butt-lift was a last minute
addition to the day's plans. All that had occurred prior to that
procedure was a three-way verbal discussion between my father
and the Ridleys with no one else around, not even the sergeant or
giggling nurse. His good intention was to enhance the cosmetic
result for his patient; his bad error was in the omission of her
signed, written consent from the medical record. Mrs. Ridley's
deposition dumbfounded Dad and his attorneys as she fully denied
knowledge of the pre-operative verbal discussion pertaining to
butt-lift. The lead defense attorney on the insurance carrier's
payroll repeatedly asked Charity Ridley about that consultation,
and she stuck to her story. Their anger over her perjury was
misdirected. Charity Ridley had been served enough of the surgical
center's complimentary wine that she had no memory of certain
blocks of time from that unfortunate day.

Cordell Pixler, Esquire, seized upon this weakness in the medical record, that hole in the fabric of the defense. "So you performed a procedure, an invasive surgical procedure, on a patient, a young innocent girl with her entire life before her, without asking her first, Dr. Foxworth? Well, there's no written consent in the chart and nothing in your consultation notes that you even discussed that part of the surgery with Flowers, much less received consent for the butt-lift from her or her mother, Doctor."

"Well, I talked with them both about it in detail. I even answered Mrs. Ridley's concern over any additional costs," Dad could do nothing but repeat that answer.

"Dr. Foxworth, is obtaining proper consent before cutting on someone's body to remove tissue an ethical medical standard in this state? And doesn't even a beginning medical student understand that it is routine to obtain such consent before electively operating on the human body?" Cordell Pixler's questions of my father were deliberately planned to be only rhetorical.

The same type of prodding dispensed during the pre-trail depositions was later put to my father on the witness stand and amplified by more oratory from the increasingly zealous Pixler. My mother, grandfather, and I did not miss a moment of the courtroom fireworks. At that point, I considered my formal schooling secondary, and no one argued. "Why, yes, Doctor," Attorney Pixler proposed, his sarcasm lost on no one, "even though you may be the only one in this courtroom at this very moment who completed medical school, the only one we must call Doctor, I would wager that everyone here (he pointed to each member of the jury) knows that a patient must be informed of what is going to be done to him or her in the operating room."

Cordell Pixler was a master craftsman, an actor who could turn fiery emotion on or off in the courtroom with abrupt, almost mechanical skill. As a series of tear drops formed in the corner of his right eye, Pixler's theatrics zeroed in to slaughter my father during the closing jury argument. "My dear ladies and gentleman, if Flowers Ridley had not been butchered by the unauthorized surgery to her buttocks on that fateful day, this bloodletting would not have occurred. Our expert witnesses have testified that if Dr. Foxworth had injected epinephrine into the tissues of poor Flowers, her bleeding might have been controlled. Dr. Foxworth himself told us up there on that stand," Attorney Pixler pointed dramatically, "that he always, yes, he said *always* injects epinephrine into those areas before he begins to slice. But, yet, there is nothing written in the patient's operative record to that effect. So we must assume that it was not done. I guess he just forgot – just forgot.

"Undoubtedly, as our experts have testified, Dr. Foxworth punctured the blood vessels lying in that very private area, punctured them like throwing darts at water balloons. Well, I ask you: would anyone expect a qualified plastic surgeon to puncture vessels in muscles to the point that a patient nearly bleeds to death?" The vehement attorney paused longer than for a routine question. "Yes, that day at the good doctor's swanky plastic surgery compound was promised to be a fresh beginning for that sweet, intelligent, innocent girl, the pride and joy of her longsuffering mother – a mother who was a mere schoolteacher only trying to do the best for her daughter by improving her self-image. The now childless Mrs. Charity Ridley spent her life's savings for her baby, an unsuspecting teenage girl."

Cordell's voice was racked with passion as he swooped down for the kill, the emotion carrying throughout the courtroom. "As a result of this, this doctor's zeal, this doctor's mistakes, Mrs. Charity Ridley has nothing left: no money and no daughter. She might as well have died right there on that kitchen floor with Flowers!"

The entire courtroom was hushed, motionless at that point in the trial, except for the stenographer who paused during typing to dab her wet eyes with a tissue.

"Let's stop and think this whole thing through once again, my friends. Just stop for a moment, clear your minds, and put this all together," Pixler pushed on after composing himself, each index and forefinger pressing against the corresponding temple. "First, how do we even know that sweet Flowers wanted any surgery done to her posterior? Where is the signed consent? Nowhere, Ladies and Gentleman, nowhere, because it simply doesn't exist. It simply does not exist," he emphasized.

"Now, I beg you to do this one thing for me – no, not for me, but for our late, unsuspecting Flowers," Cordell pleaded. "For just a moment, simply consider the horror of this deadly situation. Consider the reality of hours and hours of surgery with piece after piece of flesh removed from that part of the body resting in your hard chairs. On top of that torture, our doctor here, someone who professes himself to be the best around, tore a blood vessel so that poor Miss Ridley hemorrhaged, her blood pouring all over her raw, macerated skin." Several jury members turned white in horror. A few others buried their faces in their hands. Still a couple of others, two men in fact, nearly vomited.

Pixler continued the performance of a lifetime. "Think back about the exhibit of the autopsy photographs; they do not lie; those pictures tell the tale." Suddenly Pixler's facial expression and oratory became apologetic as he nevertheless continued the merciless desecration of my father. "Particularly for some of you ladies and kindhearted gentlemen, I know that it was hard to stomach those autopsy reports. Certainly the photos of that gruesome, horrific surgery were almost more than God meant for any of us to withstand. But thank you for enduring the visible proof.

"The wrong committed against the deceased was so very unjust."
I prayed that Pixler would stop, but he did not. "If she had not
been in such agony from her swollen – pardon me again, Ladies
and Gentlemen of the jury – buttocks area, our poor, tender
Flowers would have been able to move around better and walk
more after the long, extensive surgery. For if Flowers Ridley had
not gone under the knife in that so very personal of areas, her pain
would not have been as severe, as debilitating, and as intolerable.
Even the good doctor over there (he pointed across the courtroom
to my pale, near-diaphoretic father squirming miserably next to
his disgusted legal defense team) would have to agree with this
probability: if poor Miss Flowers Ridley had been able to walk
without meeting the unbearable pain of her buttocks hematoma,
her chance of forming that life-ending blood clot in her lungs
would have been much, much less." I watched my father shake his
head in disagreement over Pixler's perception of the facts as others
presented to his defense discredited many points of the attorney's
lengthy oral dissertation. The true disaster to my father's medical
liability case was that Cordell Pixler was just so damn good at what
he did.

Pixler's arguments continued. "You heard testimony from
our medical expert who clearly stated that the processes for the
prevention of deadly blood clots were not in place. Yes, yes, sadly
that is true. Our precious Flowers never had a chance. She was
experiencing such intense pain that she couldn't move around, so
what else could the blood in her body do?" Lawyer Pixler asked
the question rhetorically although he stared at several jurors as
though he expected an immediate verbal answer. "The only choice
her blood had in that bad situation was to stagnate in a pool of
sludge deep in the leg veins.

"Well, and we all know and understand what happened to our
Flowers. She innocently struggled to get up off the couch and

somehow made it to the kitchen to open the refrigerator. Her mother was not there; she couldn't be! She was and still is a dedicated, hardworking schoolteacher, struggling to make ends meet, a public servant to our youth who will never know the life, the grandeur of a plastic surgeon. (The judge sustained the defense objection to Pixler's reference toward my father's financial status.) Anyway, Flowers Ridley's wonderful mother could not be there to help her daughter in those final moments as the dear, innocent girl smothered. Dear God!" Pixler redirected his penetrating stare that had worked down to the last juror wedged on the back row and instead stared pleadingly at the ceiling, folding his hands together and pushing them upward to the heavens. "Please, we beseech you, our God. Tell us somehow that the preventable, deadly clot that moved from the deceased's tender, youthful legs and blocked her lungs was not painful for her at the final moment you took that wonderful, harmless girl home. She had already suffered so greatly when Dr. Foxworth ruptured that blood vessel and let the blood pour out into her buttocks."

Pixler, not my father, had the knife now and he truly knew how to kill with it. "How can we rest until we know that hers was not a death drenched in agony? How can we rest? Oh, my Dear God!"

There was not a dry eye anywhere in the courtroom, except my father's main defense lawyer who was alternately biting his lower lip. He had seen this performance too many times before.

The medical liability judgment against Sheridan Smith Foxworth, Jr., MD, et al. was 32.5 million, the largest awarded to date in Mississippi pre-tort reform. The jubilation in the plaintiff's camp was such that they settled for an additional mere five million in punitive damages and graciously decided against pursing any manslaughter charges against my dad.

Even with the additional expert witnesses brought in from the University Medical Center in Jackson, the defense team was just as ineffective in appealing the jury's decision as it had been during the initial trial itself. During a separate judicial petition, these same representatives scored only a modest victory for my dad's cause when the total award was lowered by a whopping six million. Needless to say, the five million dollars in medical liability coverage that my dad carried plus the additional two million held on behalf of the plastic surgical center as a whole fell far short of the final 31.5 million dollars granted the plaintiff. The courts seized all of my father's personal assets, forcing Dr. and Mrs. Dan Foxworth and their high school son into bankruptcy and into their new home in Granddad's pool house. Fortunately, Dad's two hundred fifty thousand dollar retirement fund and my education accounts were exempt, although a chunk of the retirement fund was used to satisfy some of Dad's own personal legal expenses.

The plastic surgery center, its spa, and the rehabilitation center were all seized and forcibly liquidated by the court's trustee in an attempt to satisfy the jury award. Not planning to forfeit any entitlement, the triumphant Pixler Law Firm submitted to the court trustee a reimbursement request of $1,335,000 to satisfy legal expenses accumulated during the discovery, trial, and appeal stages of the suit.

Those expenses were largely the result of frequent and sometimes repetitive trips made by the plaintiff's representatives in their thorough search for the truth. To obtain expert witness depositions supporting their arguments, all types of knowledgeable authorities were included in the Pixler crew's quest: experts located throughout the United States and not just in the continental region. A plastic surgeon in Hawaii was interviewed for his opinion about the cause of Flowers Ridley's death as were others in Florida, New York, and California. The plaintiff's expert who was to testify from France had to cancel at the last moment, so his testimony was done by satellite feed.

Physicians were not the only opinionated sources sought. Pixler or one of his assistants justified several trips to Canada as research into the disposable surgical equipment used on Flowers Ridley, charging all expenses to the Ridley account. In all, eight commercial, first class air flights between Memphis and Montreal were logged in and charged to the expense column of the Ridley case. The CEO of the surgical instrument company who manufactured the equipment was more than happy to discuss any concerns with The Pixler Firm. In fact, clearing the company's name and maintaining a stable stock price was imperative to keep his bonuses coming.

The issue at hand was defense claims that flaws in the surgical equipment company's disposable operating room devices had resulted in Ridley's complications of hemorrhage and hematoma formation. Not coincidentally, Pixler and Associates concurred with the manufacturer that the equipment had worked just fine. During an ensuing meeting with one of those associates, the head of the manufacturing company practically bubbled over with information supporting the fact that his products were failsafe if utilized by trained hands – the implication being that Dr. Dan Foxworth had been careless or unqualified to use the equipment. All of those meetings were billable research hours, again charged to the Ridley file.

Non-surgical medical specialists, particularly those with expertise in blood clotting disorders, were also called upon as plaintiff's experts to assess Ridley's treatment. Much of the critical testimony and opinions were repetitive. In any event, each expert charged by the hour, divulging knowledge which could be bent or interpreted with the wind's direction. These depositions required numerous trips and hundreds of hours of legal research services.

Line by line, the Pixler firm's aggressive actions followed the contingency agreement Mrs. Ridley had signed with them as her representatives. When accepting her case, Cordell Pixler had astutely smelled blood – not that of Flowers Ridley, but my father's Foxworth, old-money blood instead. Once every dime had been squeezed out of Dad's malpractice liability carrier, liquidation of his stock portfolio, sale of his personal property, and seizure of his surgical practice assets, the amount released to the court's trustee was certainly sizeable but nowhere near the judgment that had been upheld by the courts.

The balance of the money promised to her by the jury was a token consolation to Charity Ridley while her family, including her sister Faith, seemed to relish the newfound wealth, taking numbers in line to bolster support for their victimized kin. In contrast, Mrs. Ridley would certainly have relinquished all of her court winnings to get her baby back. While during the medical malpractice trial she had transferred the majority of her feelings into anger toward Dr. Foxworth and his facility, she was nevertheless weighted with a crushing mental burden at the conclusion of the final proceedings. The remorse she felt over pushing her teenage daughter to have the elective body contouring was more than simple regret; it was churned with overwhelming depression. As a result of losing her daughter, Charity Ridley had become a being void of human emotion except that of despondency. The sudden affluence was lost on the lonely mother – although she managed to spend it.

While wealth had been awarded the Ridley family, the filing of personal and business bankruptcy was the only financial option for my father and his dependents, an action of survival that came as no surprise to anyone except the Ridley family. Charity Ridley wanted every cent due her: every penny that the jury said she deserved as a tortured, grieving mother. By implying that she was merely suing the rich, faceless insurance companies that handled the malpractice coverage for Dr. Foxworth and his surgical center, her lawyer slid Charity down a misguided path of digging into deep, bottomless pockets. In the client's simple mind, the financial reserves of those companies and the amount of insurance coverage carried by Foxworth, et al. were limitless. Just as she had considered the whole lawsuit process involving the doctor to be purely impersonal, she was ignorant of Dr. Foxworth's ultimate responsibility to cough up the millions she felt due.

Also confused in Ridley's cavernous memory were the pecuniary specifics of the representation contract she signed with Cordell Pixler. Similar to her feigned lack of recall regarding verbal authorization for Flowers' liposuction and buttocks lift procedure, she now failed to remember the fine print of the Ridley-Pixler legal contract. This selective memory was jarred severely, but not into full recognizance, when she received her portion of the winning proceeds: a significant amount but much less than expected.

Per the binding agreement between Cordell Pixler and Mrs. Charity Ridley, the court trustee first deducted Pixler's documented expenses, taking millions off the top for case preparation and trial. The remaining millions were then split evenly between the firm and Mrs. Ridley, a tidy sum that would have pleased almost anyone – unless you were Charity Ridley.

The IRS first took its share of the Ridley loot as did several down-on-their-luck relatives, some of whom Charity had never met but nevertheless regarded with great pity. With seemingly good intentions, other more entrepreneurial kin and close friends sank large chunks of the new found Ridley wealth into real estate and start-up company schemes. The only profiteers from those fated and overly ambitious plans were the relatives and suddenly ex-friends who skimmed commissions from the careless investing.

For instance, the worm and cricket bait ranches struggled financially in an over-saturated market and then were wiped out by unseasonable weather. The real estate development fared no better. A determined project that at the outset seemed a win-win situation in a hungry Florida market was to consist of luxury condominiums abutting seaside mansions, acres of high-end retail space, and miles of nature trails for joggers and bicyclists. Mrs. Charity Ridley was the major investor in the entire splendor that was to include an inland lake for freshwater fishing and skiing.

Unfortunately, property excavation for the 800 acre manmade lake unearthed a clandestine toxic waste dump of which the United States Environmental Protection Agency took a dim view. To protect the waters of the Gulf of Mexico and the surrounding locale, the authorities then invoked a court order sealing the spot from development. The doomed multi-disciplined resort then alternately became a dump site for much of Charity's money. Ridley's pursuit of suing somebody and anybody over the messy land deal was diverted by the hurricane which decimated the area further, sinking more chunks of Charity's money all the way to the bottom of the Gulf, never to resurface.

Providentially for the grieving mother, she had used pre-investment funds to purchase the BMW and a new home, all with cash. The luxury automobile sat idle most of the time, filling a single garage space within her spread in Manorwood Heights of Larkspur. Now living only several blocks from my grandfather's house, Charity Ridley had never known the feeling of excessive material possessions, and for her that satiety was indeed short-lived. With her liquid portfolio having shrunk to pre-malpractice award levels because of natural and unnatural events, Charity's depression over the death of her daughter was compounded by pathological anxiety. Gone were the funds she needed to manage the overhead of her just rewards: the expensive car tag and auto insurance as well as the utilities, property upkeep, and city and county taxes that accompany a sprawling, expensive home in a high-end residential area.

During recesses from the legal proceedings, Faith Behneman had remained glued to her cell phone, creating ensembles for both daughters' upcoming beauty pageants. However, after the last court action had been completed and the malpractice award disbursed, Faith returned home to the Mississippi Gulf Coast, her share of the financial windfall in tow courtesy of her grateful sister. The portion of the jury award with which Charity had thanked her would be put to good use; Faith would be sure of it. After all the emotional support she had rendered through Flowers' death and the lawsuit and appeals, Faith considered the funds received from her sister to be heavily-deserved. The money was a handsome reward for keeping Charity propped up through the agony of losing a child while helping her to sustain the anger necessary for such a lawsuit.

"Here, this is for you," her grief-stricken sister had said as she handed Faith a chunk of the money. "I know you'll just spend this check on your girls. That's good. That's what I was trying to do: spend my money on my baby."

Spend it on her babies was exactly what Faith Behneman proceeded to do once she reached the Mississippi Gulf Coast. In fact, during the lengthy drive back home to Pass Christian, she never turned on the radio or popped in a CD. Conversely, she dreamed happily about what she could do with the money, planning systematically the shopping excursions for her daughters' pageant attire. Unlike in the past, the final selection and purchase of the wardrobes would actually be pleasurable, worryfree – no bank loan, no pawn shop needed – not this time.

And hassle-free the shopping was. After almost running to the most expensive shops, the would-be mother of pageant queens purchased multiple outfits for both daughters, using cold, hard cash – spent raw, right out of the long, bulging bank teller's envelope handed her upon cashing Charity's check.

As the excited mother promptly dumped the earlier wardrobe plans for more costly ones, the extra money created as much confusion and uncertainty as it provided varied design choices: beaded or more expensive beadless bodices, a keyhole back or maybe a deeply scooped one, real or fake leather, peacock or dove feathers.

The jewelry was another matter.

Faith had already decided that her younger daughter should try a sweetheart neckline in the next contest and the older, an empire waist. She had always wanted to see one of them in skirting of silk, and this would be the time. Through her daughters, her own flair and talents for design would emerge – at last.

Even after the revised wardrobes were finalized and purchased, Faith felt no financial constraints. Each daughter would undergo an expert makeup and hairstyle overhaul. "The pageant judges won't know what hit 'em," she bragged to herself as the proud mother doled out more cash for dance and voice lessons. She even went a step further, hiring a private instructor to coach the two. Remembering Flowers, Faith drew the line on breast implants for her second daughter although the girl undoubtedly could have used a little enhancement.

Nonetheless, after all the added coaching and removable physical amenities, Faith was certain her girls would both be knockouts on stage. No Mississippi pageant judge would be able to resist.

As Charity Ridley was agonizing over her emotional and fiscal affairs while Faith Behneman was experiencing a lifelong dream, the Foxworth family was enveloped in its own nightmare. After the malpractice trial was over and all appeals exhausted, my dad's dismal professional and financial aftermath became a reality. Following the bankruptcy, Granddad remained as supportive monetarily as Dad would allow. Senior's own suffering over our problems was silent but still deep and piercing, regardless of the fact that his son was an adult in charge of his own family.

The humiliation unleashed against my father during the malpractice trial most likely left him mentally disabled to practice medicine although he was slow to admit the weakness and consent to evaluation for such. His feelings of devastation over the verdict were not the result of any formal censure by the medical community. In fact, his previous record with the state medical licensure board was one of pristine patient care. The dismantling of my father's self-confidence came from within, fueled by the success of Cordell Pixler's actions touted by the plaintiff's camp as "nothing personal" but nevertheless perceived that way. For that matter, it was a rare physician in Mississippi or anywhere else in the United States who had never had a malpractice accusation placed against him or her.

My dad had erred not in the excessive bleeding associated with the girl's surgery because it was quickly and properly controlled, but instead in the careless omission of written informed consent – a fortunate oversight for the Pixler team and one for which Dad could never forgive himself. No matter how noble, my father's intentions to perform some of the young girl's procedures gratis had gone terribly awry, and because of that, Dan Foxworth, MD, became his own most critical, negative judge. While the jury had not done so, my dad accepted the congenital defect in Ridley's blood clotting mechanism as the ultimate cause of her untimely death. Even with that realization, he endured insurmountable anguish as well as uncertainty about his own cognitive abilities to render appropriate treatment. Those psychological doubts pushed him to question even his most basic thought processes despite the continued encouragement of his colleagues.

Dad was not alone emotionally during the medical liability trial or during its aftermath. Whether in the courtroom or attorneys' offices, Kathleen Foxworth was steadfast in her support. Mom busied herself with the intricacies of the legal procedures, continuing to shun her bridge club members and tennis team matches out of an obsession over the detail of Ridley versus Foxworth. My mother's fear of overhearing careless comments about her husband's mess was another reason, perhaps the main one, for her seemingly self-imposed social exile. However, much of her separation from society did not originate with her. She had forced herself into believing that she no longer missed or needed the festive couples' parties, the invitations to which dwindled rapidly as the Flowers ordeal blossomed.

During the malpractice trial as well as during the appeal, my mother had gently offered suggestions – gentle, at least in the beginning – in response to her husband's sounding-off episodes of frustration. Initially those exchanges had not been arguments. But once it was clear to all parties that reversal of the verdict was impossible, the ordeal was over. There was no outside enemy to defeat, only Dad's internal defeatist mentality. Other than to him, it had become obvious to everyone that Mom wanted to move on, count her blessings, and resurrect her family life. She could not easily accept my father's decision not to resume medical practice even though his insolvent partners had successfully re-established their own practices in other states.

Although my mother was not free of disappointment, she never complained about our confinement to Granddad's pool house, an area considerably more compact than her auctioned-off former home. The closeness of the new living conditions, however, provided slim privacy for personal discussions, particularly when my parents engaged in intense, screaming differences of opinion regarding management of our dismal financial situation.

Fortunately for me, I had earned a driver's license by that time and used my sixteenth birthday present to escape the lack of domestic tranquility, common in our dramatically scaled-down home. The used Jaguar was compliments of Granddad Foxworth and allowed my escape from the parental arguments, even if simply to ride around Larkspur alone.

Through loving perseverance my mother eventually won her battle in convincing Dad to get needed emotional help. She persuaded him to accept that he was clinically depressed and decaying from within and that his own family medical history could be a precipitating factor. Unknowingly, he then shared that disease with Charity Ridley, the common denominator for the cause of both illnesses being the death of young Flowers.

By then Alzheimer's disease had moved to its final stages in my only living grandmother, and Dad seemed to want to recapture his own sense of awareness, sometimes seeing himself in his mother. Finally, the no longer invincible Dan Foxworth, MD, agreed to see a psychologist, who promptly recommended the involvement of a psychiatrist.

As the shrink promised, the Vasapene was an effective antidepressant. With each bedtime dosage, Dad seemed to become less obsessed with his quandary, less anxious about the future. After a few weeks he seemed to require fewer dosages of antacid for what he described as recurring gastroesophageal reflux stemming from his stressful ordeal. His improved mental tranquility transformed the entire emotional environment of our house, our pool house. Staying home at night became much more pleasant for me as the arguments between my parents diminished.

They started socializing again, though modestly at first. After all, my Dad still had no earned income and had declined to pursue the benefits of his disability policy. Psychiatric illness would have been the disability claim, and his decision not to take up that argument reinforced my belief that in the near future Dad planned to work again.

Graceful recovery from bankruptcy was not possible for our family of three since before the Ridley incident no effective estate planning was in place for Dan Foxworth, MD. Conversely, we did have access to another tier of family money that was an advantage not afforded to most in similar predicaments. Lending the pool house to us rent-free was only the beginning of Senior's benevolence to his only brood. Granddad assumed my private school tuition expenses, and new cars for each parent mysteriously appeared. The monetary support to each of us certainly went beyond the legal annual gift limitations dictated by the IRS.

As my father's depression responded to medical treatment, a certain level of normalcy returned. Dad resumed interest in his family, turning first to my mother. His appreciation for her steadfast support was obvious through encouragement of her return to church and social activities beyond simply being a school homeroom mother. Seeing them attend couples' Sunday school again was also comforting. Composed of a high percentage of doctors and friendly lawyers, their longtime class at Larkspur Presbyterian welcomed my parents back as though they had never left. It was then that my dad casually mentioned his persistent reflux to a gastroenterologist classmate, who promptly suggested a medical workup.

Having refused the dwindling numbers of social invitations once Dad's medical liability nightmare began, Kathleen Foxworth had also let herself go, but only physically. As the court seized most of her jewelry, except for a few pieces that had belonged to her mother (that emerald ring and diamond bracelet had never been officially itemized in any joint net worth or insurance document), she had lost interest in her appearance – although her emotional strength far outlasted that of my father. Outwardly, Kathleen Foxworth had become ordinary to her husband, and for the first time since he had met her at Vanderbilt, he saw her as such. More than any other aspect of his financial, professional, and personal loss, he found the degrading physical transformation of his wife to be the most painful.

Accordingly, Mom's need for a refurbished look and a new ensemble was pressing since she and Dad had decided to attend a party in New Orleans, hosted by an old buddy from medical school and scheduled for a few weeks later. With much chagrin, the friend had closely followed Dad's devastating trial and fruitless appeals and hoped inclusion in one of his elaborate Garden District festivities would help to ease the pain.

Deciding who was more thrilled to be attending the diversion, Kathleen or Dan, was not easy. While the money likely trickled down from Granddad, it was obvious to me that Dad took great pleasure in treating his wife to a physical makeover in anticipation of the trip. To that end, the services of Minor Leblanc were a surprise. A sought-after and highly-thought-of personal stylist, shopper, and wardrobe consultant from nearby Montclair, Leblanc had been commissioned several years earlier by Mom after learning of his talents from another doctor's wife. Recognizing the need for my mother to pay some special attention to herself, Dad found Leblanc's name in an old Rolodex and called him. Through Leblanc's confidential services, my bankrupted mother would acquire what she needed, tastefully and discreetly.

"Hey, Doc! It's good to hear from you again. Of course, I remember you." Dan Foxworth had never personally met or dealt with Minor Leblanc, other that to write him a check.

Once he arranged the Leblanc surprise for my mother, Dad made sure he was not around when the stylist came calling. Since I had no warning, I was still at home on the afternoon when Minor arrived at the pool house with overflowing shopping bags.

"Just look at you!" Leblanc heaped on the compliments as soon as his resurrected client greeted him at the front door. "Not everyone can have such beautiful, thick red hair like you, Miss Kathleen, or such gorgeous ivory complexion.What a standout!" My mother stood there in shocked surprise. I doubt if she had heard anything Leblanc had said up to that point. "There's no redhead anywhere around here as fabulous as you," he smiled widely, while softly clasping his hands together.

Mom ushered him in, and the stylist walked immediately to the central living area as though a frequent visitor, freely placing all of his gear on the sofa as the packages spilled down onto the Stark rug. "When I saw this, I had to scream," Leblanc announced excitedly when he removed the first article, without question an expensive satin blouse, cut tight at the waist. His exclamation of 'This was a second scream!' introduced the coordinating skirt, which he proudly lifted from deeper in the bag. I felt embarrassed for eavesdropping, but the presentation was nevertheless entertaining. Since my mother's facial reactions were hidden from me, I wondered if she was keeping a straight face while intently studying the treasures. From my position around the corner, I was able to catch a glimpse of the artist himself as he pulled out one expensive-looking item after the other, using heavily-ringed fingers that were much too slender and well-manicured.

"Look at this jacket. Just look at it: so beautiful, so fabulous. Seeing and touching this wonderful thing brings me to tears. Do you have any tissue?" Minor continued in not-so-rare form.

"There's one last thing – for now that is. This will look great on your flight down to New Orleans, and you'll be ready to shop at

Sak's as soon as you get there." Leblanc presented another outfit, this time a black cotton car coat with a white ruched top. "And these great-fitting jeans will just set off the black boots. Sharpest outfit in the French Quarter! Yes, Miss Kathleen, wheels up!" he pronounced as he placed all the pieces together, draping them across a chair in proper order.

"Oh, I almost forgot. We will go to Candie's Closet at the mall and look for a foundation to go under this blouse," he suggested while producing the top to the next set of treasures. The presentation truly was not over. "Isn't this wonderful?" he asked, not dreaming of anything but the pleased agreement he received. "Yes, a wonderful turquoise blue twisted V-neck top," he answered himself as Mom smiled. Indeed it was an unparalleled fashion show, the best.

"For sure we will go to Candies," he stressed, his eyelids flickering out of sync. "You see ... I know my foundations." With that declaration I removed myself from earshot. I just couldn't listen to the drivel anymore although I wished that some of my dates would wear similar ensembles.

Over the ensuing days and weeks, the atmosphere around the pool house seemed to be improving. Dad had even taken up golf again, playing occasionally with Granddad's Saturday group at the Country Club. Outwardly, Senior had suppressed his own distress over the destruction of Dad's medical practice and financial stability. The stoic strength he portrayed even in the face of his son's ordeal was admired by others in the moderately-sized community, so intimate that generations of families still remained tightly knitted.

Late one afternoon after football practice, I again eavesdropped (a practice that generated less and less shame each time and one which I soon perfected), hearing Dad and Mom's debate over his continuing to remain unemployed and not collecting disability. Even though he had been mentally incapacitated by clinical depression but had rebounded with treatment, Mom and I knew that Dad's stamina and drive, both physical and mental, could be resurrected, providing he continued his antidepressant medication. Depending on Granddad for financial handouts was an unhealthy arrangement that could not remain permanent. At least that was what Mom, Granddad, and I hoped, and we believed that my father deep down felt the same.

Sooner than expected, Dad seemed to show greater interest in his own future and that of his family, an improvement which included revival of his surgical career. Not coincidentally, as I reasoned later, Senior had shared an update from the nursing home regarding his own wife's rapidly deteriorating health. My assumption is that Dad did not want to be remembered by his peers as a "head case," as was my grandmother's unfortunate distinction around town.

As time passed, I continued with high school athletics and studies and girlfriends while my parents' private discussions focused on reestablishing a Foxworth medical and surgical practice – one much less grandiose than the defunct Foxworth Center for Cosmetic and Surgical Body Enhancement. The problems they faced with that enterprise came as no surprise. Despite the pristine pre-Ridley reputation of Dan Foxworth, MD, the area lending institutions looked negatively on his personal and corporate bankruptcy. Each time my father approached even a familiar bank officer, the official would negotiate only upon the condition that my wealthy grandfather co-sign the note. Those demands for continued financial support from his own father were humiliating and degrading to the proud, once successful son. Nevertheless, my dad eventually yielded to the monetary backing of his loving, regretful, likewise tormented father.

Chapter
11

◆◆◆

THE OAK AND THE ROSE GARDEN

Having been wisely titled in the name of the eldest Foxworth, the twin engine Beechcraft Baron survived the carnage of my parents' bankruptcy. The plane was housed at the Larkspur airport, located not far from the school and convenient for Dad to pilot us on short vacations, more distant locations left to the commercial airlines. Another possession spared from the guilty malpractice verdict was Dad's pilot's license. Instrument rated since high school, he had not flown since Flowers Ridley died but resumed the passion about the time he decided to reenter other aspects of the outside world. After a few refresher, but in-depth, flight lessons down in Jackson, he was ready.

The short air junket to the Garden District soirée and the rest that New Orleans had to offer presented not only an opportunity for a long weekend getaway for my parents but also a chance for Dad to break back into flying solo. Mom was thrilled at the prospect of appearing in public with nice people, attractive out-of-town individuals ignorant of the particulars of the Foxworth family. Kathleen Foxworth was sure that she would resume her place in society, this trip being a trial run leading to a triumphant reemergence into the local social order. The last years had been difficult, a blow to her husband's self-esteem which was interlocked with her own.

Although she felt positive about her refurbished outward appearance, all to the credit of the discretionary talents of Minor Leblanc, she hoped that socializing with a fresh set of upper crust people would rebuild her inner confidence as well. The personal stylist's work with Mom in anticipation of the quick trip to New Orleans had impressed both my father and me, particularly as we witnessed her renewing self-confidence that paralleled Leblanc's swelling bank account balance.

"Dan, from what your dad says, it doesn't sound like your mother is in very good shape at all," Mom remarked as they were packing for the upcoming jaunt to New Orleans.

"Yeah, I'm concerned she may not be with us much longer. However, there is one bright aspect about her condition."

"What's that?" Mom asked as she folded the new Candie's Closet negligee selected by Leblanc. As she placed the garment gingerly into her travel bag, she sniffed to make sure it did not hint of Minor's cologne.

"Her mind's been gone for so long that she probably has no idea of what terrible physical shape she's in – completely oblivious to how fast she's going down. You know, mother always took such pride in her appearance."

"That's just so sad," Kathleen Foxworth whispered under her breath, trying to find solace in that at least the rest of her small family retained good physical health and that her husband was near total recovery from clinical depression. "Dan, this might be a good time to visit her. Couldn't we stop off on the way to New Orleans?"

"I was sort of thinking the same thing. The Madison airport is real close to Ridgeland, where the nursing home is, so I might be able to coax the St. Catherine's limo service into picking us up at the airfield. That arrangement would be a lot simpler than landing down in Jackson. Anyway, getting clearance to land the Baron in Madison shouldn't be a problem. All I have to do is submit a modified flight plan before we leave Larkspur International Airport." They both laughed at the gross exaggeration.

My parents' levity about their local airport was in stark contrast to their remorse over Memaw's physical and mental deterioration. The legal and financial troubles in Larkspur had distracted Dad from worrying about his mother while Mom's own preoccupation with the dissolution of our lifestyle had kept her from being of any help to her mother-in-law. Both of my parents counted on Granddad to attend to his own wife's needs. At some point everyone had sensed my grandmother's eventual and forthcoming demise, as is usually assumed the moment a nursing home comes into the picture.

The planned stopover in Ridgeland before continuing on with their pleasure trip was my parent's effort toward addressing that concern. Since the nurses were reporting that Memaw was fading by the minute, there was an urgent need to clear the conscience. Of course, since Memaw's degree of Alzheimer's debilitation was variable, it was likely that she would fail to recognize my parents at all, making their visit all the more one-sided. No doubt during their short morning drive from the poolhouse to the Larkspur airport, Mom and Dad discussed that possibility.

"Hello, Dr. Foxworth, your plane is being pulled up from the hangar. If you'll give us just a few more minutes, it'll be ready," reassured the manager of Larkspur Regional Airport as Dad checked in at the counter and Mom went to the ladies' room. "I'm sorry for the delay, but we're a little shorthanded. One of the mechanics – his wife went into labor early this morning – so he's at the hospital with her. It's their first baby, you know, and I hated not to let him be with her."

"Oh, I understand. No problem. We just need to get to New Orleans by late this afternoon. You see, I had hoped to have enough time to stop off on the way to check on my mother. She's in a nursing home not far from the Madison airport."

Wanting to avoid any confrontation with a much-needed customer, the Larkspur airport manager skirted his scheduling error. "I'll have you underway in no time," he stretched. Considering the state of his own elderly mother, the manager felt even sleazier about delaying the Foxworths. He had misunderstood the date my parents had planned to use the Beechcraft Baron and instead had scheduled routine service maintenance for the twin engine plane – the whole gaffe now further compounded by the airport's being short-staffed. "Monroe, hurry up with that plane in number 8," he practically yelled into the counter intercom once Dad had turned away to walk to the waiting area.

The nagging chest discomfort suddenly flared as my father patted his chest in response. "I guess I ought to have that endoscopy for this reflux," Dad muttered almost absentmindedly to the manager as he opened the morning newspaper and popped a self-prescribed Nexium from his pocket.

"Hell, I should've called in sick today, too, or gotten my girlfriend pregnant so I could get a little time off," Monroe Tuggle cursed in vain over in the hangar, where he had been the only one to show up for work as an airplane mechanic. "That ass at the front desk needs to quit pushing paper and stick his precious, perverted hands back here in this grease," he lashed out to the left engine of the Foxworth plane as he adjusted the replacement vacuum pump that was hurriedly installed the day before. The old vacuum pump had overheated secondarily to a timer malfunction of the pneumonic deice boots, the valves of which had stuck in the inflate mode but had not yet been repaired. Tuggle had worked on a similar plane a few days ago with comparable problems but, anyway, it was summer and deicing was rarely a problem. In his disgruntled, distracted state, the airplane mechanic unknowingly transposed completion of those same corrections to the plane before him as he falsely completed the repair checklist mounted to his clipboard.

"Everything's ready, Dr. Foxworth," the manager shortly announced to Mom and Dad as he escorted them to the Baron, positioned for taxi by the still-disgruntled Monroe. The manager carried my dad's small overnight bag out to the plane for him but had summoned Tuggle to carry my mom's case, which predictably was twice the size.

"All gassed up and ready to go, folks," he added as Dad stepped up on the low right wing to enter the plane. "Ya'll have a nice trip. And we got your revised flight plan all taken care of, Dr. Foxworth," the manager graciously continued while helping Mom up to the door, relieved that the Foxworths were finally on their way and showed no signs of irritation.

Watching Mom move back to nestle into one of the rear seats and continue reading her book, the manager waited as Dad closed and latched the door. The novel and its tale of convoluted murder in the Deep South had engrossed her during the last few days, with its climax approaching just as they were called to the plane. Drenched in the mystery without missing a word of text, I'm sure Mom never noticed Dad take another antacid or two as he turned on the plane's master and magnetos switches.

"This is N-2565Delta. Call for clearance delivery," Dad radioed the ground control.

"Six-five-Delta, cleared to New Orleans, Louisiana, by way of Madison, Mississippi," the controller responded in a short-winded voice strangely similar to that of the airport manager.

Typical of Mom's response to an intriguing fiction read, her pulse was sure to have quickened at the same moment that Dad's building excitement was based in reality. He had missed flying solo and was glad to have been recertified. Piloting a plane had always been a thrill for him, a total diversion from his worries, a lofty escape. I had hoped that the day would be a release for him, that he would have already begun to sense the heat of the quick-firing spark plugs designed to crank the left engine. Likewise, pushing the mixtures forward to full rich and activating the starter button would have excited him while the propeller turned four or five blades.

Removing his finger from the starter, the popping sound should have been pleasing to him. His voice was smooth and gratified when 'There's the green' was picked up by the cockpit voice recorder as the first audible speech of the flight. He had spotted the green of the indicator on the oil gauge, giving the go-ahead to start the right engine and release the parking brake. Dad could have changed the radio frequency to tower control but there was none at the bare-bones Larkspur airport, so instead he once again radioed the ground control: "This is N-2565Delta. Permission to taxi."

"Permission to taxi, six-five-Delta." The airport manager again tried to disguise his voice as controller, again unsuccessfully.

Beginning to taxi toward the runway, my father's chest discomfort apparently returned because he said aloud to himself, "This damned reflux – need to call next week and schedule that damn endoscopy." He continued in a sarcastic tone, "Great! I don't any have anymore Nexium." Even though the medication was intended for once daily dosing, like most non-compliant patients he probably hoped that doubling up would help the returning chest pain.

My mother's voice was in the background. "Check your pockets again. Don't you have at least one more in there? I looked in my purse, but came up blank. Sorry, Baby."

"I did check my pockets. Found just a couple of Rolaids." You could almost hear him chewing the chalky pills as he called back to Mom, "Kathleen, do you have your seatbelt on?"

"Yes, I'm checking the clasp now, but don't interrupt me. I really need to stay with this book. The nurse is about to get it in the bathtub – with a knife, I mean." The takeoff noise typical of our plane in its midlife crisis was beginning to mask their voices. "Dan, I'm going to put in my earplugs now. This old plane is so noisy."

Likely with the knowledge that she could no longer hear, he responded, "Well, I guess you've got all that you need back there: a great novel, a headrest pillow, and a Diet Coke."

"Ladies and gentlemen, we're at the end of the taxiway for a run-up to 1500 RPMs. Next, your captain will turn the magneto to left and right and run up the engine to 1800. And I see that the prop is doing just fine." I cried while listening to that part of the black box recording, mostly because I was happy that my father seemed to be enjoying himself. "Next, we'll set the altimeter to 550, which, ladies and gents, is the field elevation typical for northern Mississippi, and then follow with a directional gyroscope setting at 180 degrees to the south." I'm sure that he took comfort in reviewing those rote maneuvers, recently relearned during his pilot's recertification. "Co-pilot, please verify the operational status of the aileron by turning the yoke to left and right. Oh, never mind. I'll do it myself since you're still reading that book. But thanks anyway!" he laughed.

Then he lowered his voice, back to himself. "This reflux is really bad," he said quietly. "I know I'm a little anxious and excited about flying but ... " I couldn't make out the end of that sentence, but he soon resumed his playful treatise. "Passengers, we can see from the fuselage that the flaps are responding; they lower and raise nicely." Returning to a more serious demeanor with a request to turn the plane to heading 180 degrees and move down the runway,

Dad formally radioed, "Larkspur ground control, ready for take off on one-eight."

"OK, six-five-Delta, cleared for take-off. Have a safe trip." The airport manager/controller answered almost without looking up from his paperwork.

A relatively compact airport even by regional standards, the runway terminated at an adjacent section of protected, forested wetlands. By now my mom likely was fully intrigued by the quagmire of fictional plots and subplots contained within the final pages of her novel, as Dad pushed forward on the throttles with his right hand, moving the Beechcraft Baron to full power.

Knowing that the plane then began to race down the airstrip toward its own airborne climax, I have maintained hope that my father felt thrilled in returning to flying. However, knowing the detailed, assiduous man who had begun to resurface, I fear that his mind remained cluttered with the previous years of turmoil; there was no way he could ever remained focused entirely on pleasantries. Even at that moment on the airstrip, his thoughts were sure to include Flowers Ridley and her surgery – a mixture of procedures that he had performed more times than he could count, all with a track record of pleasing, safe outcomes – that is, before he was exposed to the Ridley family, the epicenter of his downfall. Listening to the silence of the voice recorder during those seconds, I could sense his reliving the weeks of court proceedings, the exact words of the dead girl's mother coming to him: her bone-chilling description of the heart-stopping horror suffered when she found her innocent daughter motionless on their kitchen floor.

I fear that at that moment his thoughts had begun to spin much like the plane's prop, except that his mind was revolving with regret and with *if only*'s. Perhaps Dad could not see the rolling runway before him but instead envisioned only the shocked faces

of the malpractice trial jury. Row-by-row, one-by-one sat the
stunned assembly of his peers, mesmerized – each overwhelmed
by the mother's gut-wrenching testimony.

"Gosh, my chest is hurting more," the recording abruptly
revealed, as he almost certainly felt nauseated. Despite being
nearly midway down the strip at increasing speed, Dan Foxworth,
MD, likely had begun to relive the courtroom drama of Ridley vs.
Foxworth: juror number three shaking her head in disgust over the
'inadequate' medical care rendered; the popping lips of a dramatic
Attorney Pixler in profile; the desperate lead defense attorney
thumbing through his notes for an impossible rebuttal; the
presiding judge nodding in agreement with the plaintiff's expert
witness that the standard of surgical care had been abandoned; the
court reporter stopping to file her nails as though the destruction
of a medical career was business as usual; and the drain of dear
Kathleen's facial color to beyond pale when the dismal verdict was
read, leaving only dark circles under the eyes of a once beautifully
exuberant wife. The most dramatic scene, perhaps, was the
pitiful-looking, tortured, middle class mother, clearly a true-born
actress, who played her part from a destroyed soul as she cried on
the witness stand and led the jury foreman to read: 'Guilty.' I can
imagine Dad's shaking his head in disgust over the tragic patient
death for which he had still not believed himself totally responsible
and his wanting to pound his fists on the plane's instrument panel
out of continued, overwhelming frustration with the outcome.

There was a background sound identified by an FAA official as
my dad's sudden opening of the cockpit mount box. Perhaps he
was searching for more antacids, remaining convinced that the
origin of his chest pain was gastrointestinal, not cardiac. "Here
they are," he sounded relieved, as I imagined him to bite off over
half the roll of antacids as the streaks of asphalt churned below the
speeding plane. Why he did not abort the flight at that point, no

one has ever understood. Nevertheless, at that moment the flight recorder revealed that the Baron was reaching 90 mph and that the nose had begun to rise toward liftoff, requiring Dad's attention.

"Have a safe trip, Dr. and Mrs. Foxworth," the manager announced over the radio as a feeble public relations gesture. He had decided to run back out to the tarmac and watch the liftoff as the plane was later shown to have accelerated to nearly 110 mph. I'm sure that Kathleen Foxworth was turning her pages fiercely, concentrating on the words and lines in her hands, her world far from Larkspur Regional Airport. Instead of pages of fiction, the Dan Foxworth I knew was recalling his family's emotional pain as his own physical, chest pain intensified. I wonder if he was crying there in the cockpit of the Baron, shedding tears of regret impossible to separate as belonging to the Ridleys or the Foxworths.

Mom had to have sensed something out of the ordinary. She was always so empathetic, always a mother, and no doubt to Dad, always a wife. During happier times when we flew the Baron as a family, long before Flowers Ridley, I remember Mom's typical glance up from her book du jour as the plane approached the last section of the runway. If she had done the same that day, she would have casually looked out the window, still in deep thought about her reading material. A one-hundred mile-an-hour blur of barren terrain would have been to her side, broken only by an occasional volunteer shrub scattered among the airport markers. She would then have looked reflexively toward my father in the cockpit, the trusted pilot, and out of the blue felt the urge to say *I love you*. But in that noisy Baron, hearing her from the cockpit was always impossible.

Monroe had joined his manager at the ground facility. "Wonder what's making that guy take so long to lift off?" the puzzled, but worried, mechanic asked weakly.

From the location of the skimpily numbered airport personnel, the plane's acceleration seemed purposeful, but delayed. Dad's concentration on the liftoff procedures was surely renewed with an adrenaline surge, his fists clenched around the main control with a forceful grasp of agitation laced with guilty frustration. I have imagined that he then released his fist to grasp again the yoke with such force that my mother would have been surprised, concerned that he planned to pound himself against it.

"Dunno, Monroe. Gave him clearance plenty of time ago. I was just getting ready to radio him again when he lifted off. He must be late in pulling back." The two men followed the forward lifting motion of the plane, much like following a thrown football, their eyes dramatically meeting the oak and pine trees ahead of the aircraft at the end of the runway. For my dad those oak and pine trees must have appeared from nowhere, rising out of the marsh as the runway disappeared under the nose of the plane, jolting Dan Foxworth, Jr., MD, back from the Larkspur courthouse where he had lost everything.

Oblivious to the Foxworth saga, Monroe pulled his left hand back toward the side of his waist, hoping that Dr. Foxworth was doing the same. However, I feel sure that at that second Dad hoped that he could lift Mom and himself (as well as me) above the world and its weight, his left hand pulling the yoke back sharply, demanding enough for liftoff while the right handled the throttles and started to raise the landing gear.

"Shit, he'll barely miss the tops of those tall pines!" Instead of the accelerating Beechcraft Baron before him, Tuggle unexpectedly saw a mental image of the clipboard he had left suspended on a nail in the mechanics' hangar. The sloppily completed checklist of the Foxworth repairs throbbed before him, the bold print provoking shame for the careless and hurried inspection.

As I listened to the last moments from the black box, I could sense Dad's instinctive, renewed catecholamine surge that would force him to jerk harder against the controls, in fruitless human effort. Suddenly there would have been no feeling in his left arm along with crushing, unbearable chest pain. The recorded cockpit sounds remained void of human noises although I can imagine Dad's glancing back down to the yoke, and then forcing his right hand to cross over to relieve the paralyzed left. The flight data would show that he had not fully pulled the landing gear up, and with this faltering at the finish of the runway, the plane never reached full power. Ninety-five mph was adequate rotation speed to raise the nose, but fell well short of proper liftoff speed. The moment that the Beechcraft Baron needed more momentum, my dad could no longer have had the strength to control the pull-back, no strength to force more power to the engines.

The FAA speculated a heart attack. Since heart attacks can present in different ways, I have clung to that possibility, most certainly the rarer cardiac vasospasm variety since Dad wasn't much for fried food and did not have elevated cholesterol or high blood pressure.

Loss of consciousness from a heart attack, for example, would result in Dad's falling as far backward in the pilot's seat as the restraints would allow, which I was told by the investigators would result in a natural pull-back against the controls. Strangely, that action must have been more effective than any of his preceding purposeful efforts.

The manager of our small airport and his trusted mechanic watched in disbelief as the top of a sixty-year-old pine tree was a narrow miss for the Foxworth Baron as the right engine smashed the first oak off the runway. An eighty-year-old trunk then took out the prop, causing the craft to shake violently out of balance.

The Baron reached 150 mph but flew only in cartwheels as the plane was seen to clip more trees like a ball bouncing across a baskctball court. The autopilot engaged and disengaged itself inconsistently, the uncontrolled maneuvers accompanied by the sharp, panicked screams recorded from my mother, "Dan, Dan, what's wrong? Are you all right?" In her final moments, Kathleen Foxworth thought only of her husband. From her seat she could have seen that he sat unconscious, his drooping head shifting from side to side with the erratic movements of the plane.

Mom had never piloted an airplane, but certainly she could have decided to try. However, in unbuckling her seat to move forward, the fruitless effort would have been overcome by the nausea and vomiting of disorientation. There was evidence of a sound within the fuselage as though a body, her body, had fallen against the cabin side panel, striking it violently enough to snap her head sideways.

Had my parents been conscious, they would have seen the Mississippi terrain spin by like a carnival ride, heading back into the nearby city limits of Larkspur. Moving as if on impulse, the aircraft rolled sharply to the left as it descended deeply and uncontrollably. The Baron began to undulate violently as it spun nearly to a fully nose-up position. During the next few seconds, it rotated far enough right and back left to follow with a full three hundred sixty degree spin to almost level off.

As though clairvoyant, Gregory Whitestone glanced out the closed side window of his headmaster's office. On impulse he threw back his leather chair and dove headfirst into the foot space under the desk, squeezing to a snug fit. His vision was of my parents' plane plummeting out of control as it tumbled in a rollover without the benefit of a conscious pilot. Quickly covering the short distance between the airport and the school, the plane flipped across the airspace of the campus as it passed over the parking lot and clipped a row of prized oak trees. After narrowly missing Whitestone and the administration building as well as the adjoining football stadium, the plane crashed in a ball of fire, charring the adjacent vacant field.

Fortunately for the school, the crash occurred during the week of an away football game, giving the high school several days to shore up the minor tree damage and camouflage the gruesome plane wreckage before hosting the next match. Despite the importance of appearances to alumni and parents and until the investigation of the accident was completed, Whitestone's cleanup crew was prohibited from clearing the charred, mangled debris from the field. As a result, the band and cheerleaders were forced to practice elsewhere.

The funeral visitation was Friday and the burial services the next afternoon. Because my parents had died, the head football coach excused me from that away game and spared one of his assistants to baby-sit me during the visitation and funeral. The decision to do without one of his most valuable players was difficult but painless, considering that the upcoming Larkspur opponent was a notoriously pathetic team from southern Tennessee that our school annually pulverized whether playing here or there. Regardless of Larkspur's certain win in Tennessee, that Friday out-of-town football game excused the head coach from attending my parents' visitation while his prior commitment to accompany our kicker to a college scholarship interview got him out of Saturday's funeral.

The closed caskets lay side-by-side, weighting the front of our church while the crowds of mourners spread densely throughout the sanctuary were equally as heavy. Memaw had been transported to the Larkspur Presbyterian Church by ambulance, attached to an oxygen tank and flanked by nurses as she sat on the front row. Granddad was seated next to one of her attendants.

"Hey, Memaw, I love you. I'm glad to see you. Mom and Dad were on their way to check on you," I spoke softly while giving her weak, brittle frame a soft embrace. I had joined my only two close living relatives on that pew, but Memaw's blank eyes told me that she was unaware of her whereabouts and mine. Through the tears that then sprang from my myriad emotions, I could easily see the once vibrant woman who supervised the cookie baking and issued suffocating hugs of welcome to me every afternoon after school. It was impossible to forget those happy times although I realized I had become an orphan, and what was so much worse was that I was an only-child orphan. There was no one with whom to share the loss of my parents; the anguish rested within my ruptured soul. My grandfather was all that was left for me, but he was dealing with his own demons.

Despite my eyes watering enough to cause dehydration, I could still see down the pew to Granddad, wondering if he was as envious as I of his wife's oblivion. Her mental and physical condition spared her the shrinking family's great heartache. Mrs. Sheridan Foxworth, Sr., knew nothing of what the Foxworths had endured and continued to suffer.

Until that Saturday's services began, Senior's stoicism over the deaths of his son and daughter-in-law was not surprising. Although his eyes that day at the funeral did not have the same blank, hollow stare as those of his wife, they nevertheless cast a grief-stricken fog that I would see again. Fully absorbing the shock of the tragedy as the minister began the eulogy, Granddad's emotions surfaced for the first time since the Baron went down. Many admire a man unafraid to cry, but his tears were not for the others around him; they were for himself. The tears he wept that dismal Saturday merely hinted of the episodes to follow, such as when I found him later in his den with the newly archived home videos and the manuscript of Dad's graduation speech at Harvard.

The church and graveside services seemed endless. The sadness of my parents' death was rephrased in every imaginable description but mixed with hope for the future in their promising son, both an athletic standout and serious student. I kept my head buried deep in my hands during much of it, feeling a tremendous burden. Finally the ordeal was over, freeing the lucid members of the Foxworth clan to be whisked to Granddad's estate while Memaw was shuttled back to the nursing home in Ridgeland to await her own such ceremony a year later. Since a few of my grandfather's great-nephews and -nieces had come to join my maternal uncle and his family for the unhappiness, I was forced to renew acquaintances with these distant relatives in the form of dismal talk. Fortunately the compact band of cordial, grieving, distant relatives did not linger afterward. At least the mourners left well-fed, compliments of the spread laid out by the organized wives of Granddad's closest golfing buddies.

Perhaps the most surprising moment of the funeral services was provided by the audacity of Mr. and Mrs. Cordell Pixler. Certainly their motivation was more out of curiosity than respect. As the Pixlers moved through the receiving line of Friday's funeral home visitation, the stares rendered them by the other members of my small family and our friends were no match for the red glow of hatred erupting from Granddad's eyes. Only his impeccable social breeding kept him from slugging the guy as Cordell extended his sympathetic hand and Rachel Pixler tried a weak hug. In Cordell my grandfather saw the person who had destroyed his son's life – and his own.

During the lonesome, brooding weeks and months immediately after my parents' funeral, Senior was consumed with anger over the death of his only child – so much so that he could not even listen to the car radio, read a book, look through a magazine, or watch television. Around others he seemed pleasant, almost normal, occasionally laughing or joking. But alone he was a different man, thinking of nothing but the loss of his son.

Grandfather continued to go to church every Sunday, the same church in which the funeral was held, each week reliving the memorial service with renewed physical and mental anguish.

Throughout my freshman year at Ole Miss, I tried to return to Larkspur on the weekends to attend church with him. However, the eleven o'clock service was early, very early, especially for a university student who used his weekend mornings to recuperate from the drudgery of a week spent trying to catch up on coursework or recuperate from the previous weekend's parties. Between nods, I remember one sermon in which something was said about being so hurt, so angry that a person could not bring himself to pray – situations where deep inside the soul there was intense anger but also complete emptiness. The minister said that in those devastating instances the acceptance of well-wishing offers like *I'll pray for you* were important to heal that damaged, tortured heart. He explained that God would listen to those prayers from others and one day open that broken heart to recovery and understanding.

I looked over at my grandfather during that church sermon, one of few that I had not slept through using chewing gum as a successful stimulant. His head was motionless, his profile blank, his eyes foggy. True, Granddad's face and eyes were directed at the Presbyterian minister and his message, but he heard nothing at all.

Charity Ridley had lots of minutes left on her plan but spent only a couple to phone her sister that day. As she had hoped, the call went to voice mail. The would-be mother of state-winner beauty queens was busy on her own cell phone engaging a college history professor, local newspaper editor, and clinical psychologist to ripen the minds of her prized offspring. Leaving no aspect of pageant preparation to chance, particularly the scores to be earned from the judges' interviews, Faith was determined that no other entrants would be more prepared.

"It was all for nothing, Faith," Charity spoke into voicemail, as hoped. "Why couldn't I have left my baby alone? She was so smart, so pretty inside – she just didn't know it. I only wanted to bring that beauty out so that she and the whole world around her could see how truly gorgeous she really was. Was I so wrong?" Charity stared out a French door and across the backyard to the elaborate rose garden, inherited from the previous owner. As she continued with the message for her sister, she painted imaginary blossoms on the bushes in the fall landscape. "I'm so very, very sorry. There has been a great deal of tragedy and much anger." A strange smile that no one could see crossed the woman's face as she ended the call, "There's simply nothing else left for me to do now."

Tossing the cell phone into the seat of a sunroom chair, Mrs. Ridley turned almost 360 degrees in panoramic inspection of the lonely interior. Ideally, the house in which she stood would have been a lifelong dream home for most, except that it was left filled with miserable emptiness for her. Moreover, there was no way she could continue to afford the house, a mansion by most standards. She knew that her sister would not be able to afford the upkeep on it either, even considering the lawsuit money she had shared.

"Besides, Faith would never move to Larkspur; she loves the coast and all that sun too much. She wouldn't feel comfortable about living here. Knowing my sister, she'll put this place up for sale as soon as she gets it," she decided walking out onto the patio, leaving the door ajar. "That'll leave more money for her to spend on those girls – maybe that will make her feel better about everything," her melancholy voice trailed off.

Charity moved down the patio steps, past the pool, and then over to stand at the rose garden now barren of all but a few remaining leaves. "Oh, I wish they were blooming now. Flowers loved roses," she remarked as though giving a garden tour.

Adjoining the collection of antique and more modern grafted varieties was a parterre lined by low, manicured boxwoods and filled with panels of still green fall grass. While once again admiring the landscape architect's design of separate, raised rose beds shaped in natural stone, she decided for a multitude of reasons that this was the right place. She would stand among these lovely gardens, on the smooth grass of the parterre just next to the roses. The blades of green within the panels of the gardens would grow fresh again and the roses would return in the spring, erasing the residual of her despondency.

"Yes," she decided as she turned briefly to look back toward her house. "On the lawn area near the rose beds will be better. The flagstone around the pool and on the patio will stain." Likewise, Charity felt that using the inside of the house would leave an undue burden for someone.

Even though she was outside instead of behind closed doors, she felt secluded, hidden at the rear of her property and yet more alone than she could feel anywhere else. Mrs. Charity Ridley was certain that the thick shrubbery and tall trees would hide her secret for awhile. Growing along the high brick walls bordering her yard, the vegetation would complete a visual shield in addition to muffling the sound. The neighbors would know nothing, not at first. Here by the rose garden, no one would find her for hours or maybe for even longer, giving God plenty of time to take her. She searched her memory for Bible passages dealing with His word about her plan, but came up empty. This miserable soul knew that what she was going to do was wrong, except it felt so right for her, for now.

Charity first removed the wallet from her purse that she had uncharacteristically carried out into the backyard. Thumbing through the photographs in one of the folding sections, she studied her late daughter's pre-surgical face and body, erasing any doubt about her true intentions for Flowers, intentions that had gone wrong, very wrong. All she had wanted for her baby was a worldly improvement so that barriers to new experiences would be broken as the poor child developed some self-confidence.

"Maybe the doctor didn't do anything wrong, but maybe he did. Anyway, he's dead now. Was God punishing him with that plane crash?" she asked aloud, having read in detail the newspaper articles about the accident.

"Maybe God was punishing me for trying to make my baby into something she wasn't supposed to be," she resolved as she returned her wallet and the pictures to her purse. With trembling hands, she dug deeper into the bag for what she needed next and retrieved it. After inserting the handgun's metal cylinder into her mouth, she perceived the barrel as amazingly cool, tasting oily and bitter.

"Dear God, please forgive me," she spoke, holding the revolver in place. "Please let me be with my baby, my Flowers," she prayed.

The lawn maintenance service crew came to the Ridley house a few days early that week. Mrs. Ridley had ceased to pay her bill on time, and this was to be her last service call. That afternoon the public high school student who owned the maintenance service had planned to break the news tactfully: he was dropping her as a client purely out of financial necessity. Anyway, his conscience was clear. He had a waiting list of potential, better paying customers and had always done a good job for Mrs. Ridley.

For that final day, the young man had wanted to leave Mrs. Ridley's grounds in perfect shape because she had always been such a nice lady. As he did every other week, he would make sure that she received a professionally manicured yard and, as usual, would work the backyard gardens himself. He dreaded having to tell her that she could no longer be his customer, especially since her daughter had died a while back, but his college education fund needed every penny he could earn.

As the teenage entrepreneur rounded the corner of the house and entered the gate to the rear, he hoped he would not encounter Mrs. Ridley until the job was finished. He wanted to delay the unpleasant news until after he collected the final bill – in full this time and in cash since the last check bounced. Definitely feeling awkward about the situation but believing her termination to be necessary from a business standpoint, he cleared his conscience. He was desperate for the money.

About a third of the way into trimming the backyard, the awkwardness the teenager had feared in confronting Mrs. Ridley became a moot point. That afternoon near the rose parterre gardens, his unease was replaced by an entirely different emotion as he grabbed his cell and dialed 911.

The Ridley bill would go unpaid once again.

Chapter
12

•••

THE PLANS

"Where's the wine closet?"

"It's over here, off the kitchen, in easy access to the dining room," the architect answered with forced patience, reinforced by the mental arithmetic of his mounting commission.

The Pixlers had signed the customary contractual agreement for the home-design services of Hobby Dencil, the renowned Memphis architect popular beyond the confines of the immediate Deep South. Hobby had agreed to meet with the Pixlers only after they had arranged a referral recommendation from another Dencil client, also a successful attorney. Worthy individuals like the Pixlers proceeded as Dencil clients, assuming they survived the screening process: a $20,000 retainer fee before structural and design concepts were discussed, then agreement to a minimum two-million dollar construction budget. The total architectural fee amounted to a twenty percent take of the final construction cost, almost certain to balloon beyond the original estimates.

Cordell and Rachel Pixler's project was mushrooming, following the typical pathway of a Dencil Design. The need for an ever-expanding, increasingly elaborate dwelling surfaced early during the drafting process of their home. But clients like the Pixlers quickly found favor with Hobby Dencil. Within ten days of receipt, Cordell Pixler's administrative assistant satisfied every monthly invoice submitted for payment by the esteemed architect. Frequent drives between Memphis and Larkspur had been the rule for the Pixler project and all at billable hours. In fact, at one point, Cordell offered to rent Dencil a condo in Larkspur, hoping to eliminate some of the architect's travel time. Though Dencil politely declined that alternative to driving back and forth, citing the need to remain in close proximity to his draftsman in Memphis, his true reason was to minimize the time spent in lowly, tacky Larkspur.

Many Dencil-Pixler architectural design meetings were held impromptu, almost as if they were emergencies. One notable example was Rachel's acute panic over lack of china and silver space in the butler's pantry or Cordell's fear that his mahogany-paneled study was not roomy enough for all his smoking buddies and their choice cigars.

That mahogany study had been a thorn for Hobby Dencil, AIA, from the moment he met with Cordell Pixler. Never a big fan of state-of-the-art electronic conveniences (Dencil even considered a television, one with a screen large enough to see, extremely gauche), he had regretted lowering his standards to blend stereo equipment and wall-mounted plasma televisions into the home's overall decorative design. Of course, the pain was offset as both the final construction cost of the mansion and his net commission ballooned with every client meeting, scheduled or not, as additions and revisions to the original architectural scheme mounted. To Hobby's delight, the Pixlers jumped at the idea of an extensive wireless communication network to be hidden throughout the dwelling along with an equally costly, but camouflaged, computer equipment system. Hobby bore secret pride in the fact that he had satisfied the wealthy couple's fascination with twenty-first century gadgetry but had still minimized an unsightly show of modern indulgence.

Forget the practicality; even when drawing a private family dwelling, Hobby Dencil's trademark concept centered on an artistic, old world-influenced showplace of elite, but tasteful, architectural interest. The architect possessed no true interest in the technosavvy twenty-first century and included those features in his blueprints only upon client demand, but usually not without argument. His own minimal personal effort toward moving to modern electronic wizardry consisted of the recent exchange of his pager for a cell phone, albeit last year's model.

"I allowed for his and hers bathroom suites, as you requested." Dencil swallowed hard to prevent choking while revealing the next page of the bound architectural renderings. Rachel studied the diagrams intently. Cordell checked his watch.

The Pixler home was to contain unfathomable total square feet, and this majestic bathroom wing extending from the master bedroom suite befitted such a financially unburdened couple. Their limitless expectations were recognized early in the preliminary stages by Hobby Dencil, even before specific elements of design were discussed.

"Is this where the plants will go?" Rachel Pixler had always dreamed of a tropical shower, an herbal wonderland in which an outsized water haven was surrounded by thick, broad-leafed plants. Circumferential skylights and exterior glass walls opening to a secluded outside garden would illuminate the shower occupants as well as the indoor vegetation.

"Yes, and the climate controls will be located over here on this wall," Hobby responded as he directed his pointer pen toward a corner of the inked drawing. "Summer breeze ... light winter snow ... spring shower ... whatever," he choked. "You'll be able to access the controls from the oversized Jacuzzi over here." Adding with disguised disgust, "Oh, and you asked that enough space be allowed for more than two occupants in the tub. I have provided for the largest, non-commercial, indoor personal Jacuzzi available. But I left off the mirrored ceiling above it. You'll never be able to see anything for all the condensation." Hobby again swallowed hard with revulsion over his own propagation of such indulgence, his repugnance quickly suppressed in anticipation of the extra commission.

In their countless discussions held over bottles of fine wine, the Pixlers had envisioned a striking, palatial entrance to their future estate, ideally perched atop a gentle hill. The remaining obstacle was obtaining that hill in an area of Larkspur that would satisfy the discriminating Mrs. Cordell Pixler. Even after Cordell's unsuccessful real estate contacts failed to locate such suitable property, the design process forged ahead. Without argument, Hobby Dencil accepted the affluent couple's initial concept for the front of their home still on the drawing board. To that end he specified wide, lengthy sheets of Oklahoma flagstone harvested from Arkansas and crafted into an exterior staircase leading to that main entrance. That entrance would beckon one to what only the Pixlers would consider to be a majestic, architectural wonder.

Architect Dencil remained determined to restrict the Pixler project to good taste, notwithstanding its impracticality. His comfort level over the final appearance of the challenge was satisfied, at least temporarily when Cordell discovered the available Architzel property. Still concerned that the front elevation designs might be overdone but nevertheless appropriate for a large residence intended for entertaining, Dencil believed that the Oklahoma stone would blend naturally into this unexpectedly available construction site. For the first time since he had been contacted by Cordell Pixler, Hobby Dencil felt a renewed degree of self-respect for his choice of projects. Once the multi-acre Architzel tract was cleared of the charred debris, it was transformed into the choicest of locations upon which to build the vision.

This commission had now become a proud credit for the Hobby Dencil name: a mansion rising out of a piece of prime, established real estate in a neighborhood of other fine, expertly designed and built homes. Unlike so many other structures in the South and elsewhere, this mansion would blend into its surroundings as though it had always stood there, rather than as a fabrication of forced visual interest erected on a landfill. The final architectural plans for the challenging Pixler couple would not seem contrived. Dencil was sure of it.

"Six weeks, that's all it'll take. You can stay in a motel near the training center. A lot of new ones have cropped up near the airport. There's a real nice Courtyard that I stayed in one week while filling in for an instructor who had the flu. I remember it had a free hot breakfast every morning and snacks out at night. The department will pay your lodging bill – sort of a hiring bonus, you might say."

Thomas Lisenbe had wasted no time in claiming his payment for rescuing me from the clutches of Lyric Sleethe and her cronies. My rationalization of the dead-end situation was that I needed a new job anyway, and serving as a public servant through the fire department was certainly respectable, maybe more so than as a private school science teacher. Moreover, this career direction would parallel my bursting into a burning house to save an elderly woman and her dog, if only halfway successful.

Sorting through that whole scenario with the DUI arrest and my alternative to conviction, I thought about Dickens and what would happen to him during my six-week training session in Storck, much less during a prison stay. Of course, I assumed I would be free to drive back to Larkspur for the weekends while enrolled at the firefighting academy, but for all I knew, the instruction could be intense enough to bleed past Friday afternoon. Resisting the idea of boarding my yapping, adopted pet at a kennel, my humane animal instincts were upheld with Kaylee's offer to keep the aging Chinese pug for me in my absence. After all, the poor dog had already been orphaned once.

The availability of the Courtyard Motel became irrelevant because the Barracks, a period 1950s dormitory, stood adjacent to the fire academy. During my briefing, Marshal Lisenbe had conveniently forgotten about that unique lodging feature included as part of the training. The administration required its cadets to live there on campus, a facet of our education that became obvious once the nightly fire and rescue drills started. Another surprise regarding the six-week adventure was that it was indeed forty-two days, a true crash course in becoming a firefighter that included weekend classes consisting of mock fires and accident rescues.

As a result, the anticipated weekend trips back to Larkspur and Kaylee – and Dickens, of course – were impossible because the instructors reduced the length of the Saturday and Sunday class time by only a few hours. This was enough time for conjugal visits away from campus, making the nearby Courtyard Motel useful to most, but since my relationship with Kaylee had not yet progressed to that point, I was content to let her remain in Larkspur to attend to Dickens, instead of me.

Alvin Coakley was the veteran professor of the Storck Fire Training Academy, *veteran* in the sense that he had taught at the facility since its inception. He certainly would have been tenured if the distinction had existed for such institutions. Watching Coakley stand in front of the chalkboard with a belly-overhang obscuring his belt buckle, not to mention the ubiquitous white chalk streak in the crack of his trousers seat, was almost more than my sense of humor could stand without erupting. The mental picture of Professor Alvin Coakley clad in classic fireman's uniform complete with matching hardhat, holding a black water hose, was in itself comic relief for his education about fire drafts, CPR, and acute care of third- and fourth-degree burn victims.

Coakley was old-fashioned, remaining suspended in the era of chalkboard instruction, resisting power-point, overheard projectors, or even erasers for the chalkboard. In fact, he used his right hand to clean away the white marks from the board, thus the trouser streaks. From the appearance of his soft, pale hands and flushed W. C. Fields-style face, one would naturally wonder if he had ever personally fought a fire or performed any feat that required much physical exertion.

To make a long story short prefaced Coakley's customary summation of each day's lesson. In fact, the phrase was used repeatedly in each class that he taught, sometimes in the middle of an explanation to his fire-fighting neophytes even when the explanations pointed to no important concept at all. Hearing that American colloquialism in everyday conversation with others still conjures for me a detailed vision of Alvin Coakley. Al was a wealth of wisdom about exterminating raging fires and investigating their causes. Questions and interruptions to his lectures were always allowed, creating one of the most tolerant classroom experiences that I have ever had.

The master left to the more agile instructors the majority of the hands-on teaching required in the flame ignition and extinguishing labs. Those dedicated guys were not fulltime employees of the training academy, but still appeared on a scheduled basis as a challenge to the cadets. Much like exercises I had endured as a pre-med student at Ole Miss, they administered science lab practicals which, of course, skipped the dissections of fetal pig, embalmed cat, or small shark specimens but confronted us with naming fire accelerants and recognizing characteristic points of origin associated with particular blazes. There was a crossover, however, in the identification of elements within chemical compounds. While the younger instructors – that is, those in their early thirties and forties – were actually responsible for planning and putting on those informative shows, sixty-year-old Al Coakley remained in full command of the proceedings.

Ignoring the fact that a noticeable percentage of the classes was composed of females, Coakley would reaffirm with *what we're trying to do is make sure that at the end of the day you've been a good fireman,* another of his favorite colloquialisms. Whether or not it was appropriate to refer to the women cadets as firemen or to lump us all in the vernacular of *firepersons,* I was never certain. Al's use of this phrase played like a scratched CD, surfacing in nearly every conversation with him, personal as well as instructional. *At the end of the day* was to Al Coakley a summary statement of life's work effort: save lives and protect property from fire.

Our chief instructor ignored the protocol at other firefighting academies the size of Storck where training exercises were confined to extinguishing blazes and saving lives. In contrast, his curriculum was designed to push each student until the points of origin were unmasked. His dictum was that a firefighter should take charge of the scene without leaving the task to special investigators who would follow behind.

The truth was that Alvin Coakley would still have remained with the Bureau of Alcohol, Tobacco, and Firearms training staff, his first love, had he not been involuntarily removed. During that

time in Glencoe, California, the particulars of fire investigation
began to fascinate him. Not only did he find the mental exercises
rewarding, but investigating after the fact was much less exerting
than battling an engulfing blaze firsthand. Coakley kept his mind
and body clear when engaged in those investigative exercises,
but his time away from the bureau's assigned training duties was
another matter.

One weekend when Coakley was unexpectedly called to oversee
the management of an actual fire scene, he brought with him the
smell and effects of alcohol, hinting at his after-hours addiction.
He was at the time too knowledgeable to lose as an instructor and,
fortunately for the bureau, faithfully followed the requirements of
his treatment recovery and probation. As he continued teaching at
the school and participating in on-site investigations, there were
rumors of his having a little sip now and then, here and there.
Nevertheless, the innuendo was always dismissed as just that.

Truthfully, Coakley had remained sober since his treatment, but
the desire along with his employment probation persisted. His
downfall was an indiscretion celebrated with a female underling
one evening. Unaware of the anxious young woman's intentions
to advance her own career through and ahead of him, Coakley
carelessly succumbed to alcohol with her at a bar and was busted.
In all probability, Al would have been successful with his
defense of being the victim of a setup if his judges had been simply
his peers.

A panel of those peers promptly summoned Coakley to a
compact basement conference room for a probation hearing.
Held before ATF professionals in addition to other fire bureau
instructors, the stone-faced group sat lined end to end at a
conference table, waiting for him. Beginning with formal
introductions, the main adjudicator next read two passages from
the employment protocol designed to handle such issues of broken

trust. To Coakley's surprise, that chief spokesman was not one of his usually supportive crew, but instead an outsider, an aggressive lawyer out to impress everyone but the accused. The attorney portrayed the couple of after-hours cocktails as much more than a slip. Al's actions were characterized as a slap in the face of the entire bureau along with God, truth, justice, and the American way.

Immediately after the unfavorable judgment was rendered, Coakley was bounced from the school but was allowed to continue in his field under the condition of sobriety. One buddy who had served on the panel at the probation hearing kindly found Al a job at the start-up fire academy in Mississippi, where Coakley thrived and the buddy cleared his conscience.

The trip to France was a much needed diversion for the busy lawyer and his socially aspiring wife. Primarily to divert Rachel from her obsessive house planning, Cordell had suggested the getaway and immediately chose the location under the guise of continuing legal education. The cafes, boutiques, art galleries, and nightclubs in the vicinity of the Seine River were a draw to anyone with disposable income who wanted to relax and have fun in luxury. And the Pixlers certainly belonged in that category. Unfortunately for Attorney Pixler, the scheme backfired.

From a financial standpoint, Mrs. Pixler had unquestionably done well in her matrimonial match. Not only did her high profile plantiffs' lawyer husband keep a steady stream of settlements and jury verdicts coming in, but he liked to recycle the money, with Paris becoming a favorite European spot and Venice, a close second. During this particular excursion, Cordell actually attended various international legal seminars during the day, but managed

several hours of Parisian shopping later with his sensuous wife.
Jewelry was bringing its just rewards.

While the couple was staying near the *Saint-Germain-des
Pres*, Rachel first spotted a picture of the castle in a current copy
of *Marvelous Castles and Manors of Europe*. The real estate
magazine beckoned as she relaxed in an often-frequented salon
and day spa near the Hotel Le Senat. During her lengthy pedicure,
she studied the lead article in detail, noting a firm's plans to
dismantle an ancient castle on the outskirts of Paris. The one
remaining direct descendant of the original owners, a Monsieur
Simone, was quoted as lamenting the sale of the historic site to
the salvage company while attributing the property's liquidation
to economic downturns. Somehow Simone shifted most of the
responsibility for France's loss of such celebrated places to
the greedy Americans who kept the wrecking balls in business
with irresistible financial offers. Somewhere in the dialogue the
profiting owner specifically blamed President Bush for the castle's
destruction.

Ignoring the political commentary, Rachel was mesmerized by
the periodical's descriptions of the ostentatious marble Italian
fireplaces, along with the grandiose fleur-de-lis fencing and other
antique architectural remnants that would be available once
the castle was dismantled. She had never seen anything even
remotely as lavish in any house in Larkspur, over in Montclair, or
in Memphis, Jackson, Dallas, or Atlanta. Even before she had ever
heard of Cordell Pixler, Rachel had never missed an opportunity
to tour any of the extraordinary homes within driving distance.
And perpetually, there was occasion to do so. One of the private
schools or an organization like the Humanitarian Alliance or
a homebuilders' association frequently promoted some local
tour of homes, interior designer showcase, before-and-after
transformation, or the like.

There in the salon's spa Rachel melted, her toes soaking up a silky solution with an aroma that invaded the nostrils. As her decorative imagination ran rampant, page after page of exquisite objets d'art were displayed before her as the magazine catalogued the available French architectural remnants. She decided then that the carved Italian marble featured in a special section would make enviable lintels over the doors in her foyer.

Absorbing the magazine's articles as though trying to commit them to memory, she decided to permanently borrow the publication for later reference; the shop would never miss that copy of *Marvelous*. While the pedicurist stepped away for a moment, Rachel folded and then slipped the journal deep into her bag, glancing around her section of the salon to see if anyone had noticed. But no one was watching; everyone was either too busy becoming beautiful or beautifying someone else.

After reflecting on the months of architectural deliberation that she and her husband had logged with Hobby Dencil, Rachel now wanted her new house to resemble that French castle, or at least exude its magnificence. Cordell would agree with her; she was sure of it. But would Dencil? Throughout it all, her husband's desire for a truly splendid house, a magnificent, distinctive one, had been obvious. The examples in this wonderful magazine, held close in the deepest recesses of her bag, were sure to be what he wanted, what she wanted.

As the attendant returned with more scented oils, she drenched Rachel's toes and returned them to the thick water. Rachel barely noticed; she was mentally redesigning the main entrance to her planned home, rethinking it as even more opulent – far beyond the imagination of tacky Larkspur – and more importantly, casting aside the labored designs of Hobby Dencil. While in Dencil her husband had undoubtedly hired the most expensive architect he could find in the region, she was certain that Cordell would agree with her new ideas. Rachel was absolutely sure.

Convincing eccentric and opinionated Hobby Dencil would be a greater challenge; Rachel was sure of that, too. But it was possible. Although Dencil was southern-bred, his cosmopolitan mannerisms, decorative flair, and slightly affected British accent could have placed him anywhere: New York, LA, London, even Paris. Surely he would agree with her inspired house design revisions, born of Paris and the French countryside. Dencil would want to be part of the magnificent insight that Rachel and her husband would introduce into the architectural legacy of the miserable Larkspur community.

As she mentally sketched some of her ideas, Mrs. Pixler referenced what she could remember from the alluring magazine pages. A few of the desired images were becoming a confusing collage, and she longed for "her" edition of *Marvelous* tucked secretly out of sight. "I'll still need Hobby to figure it all out," she said aloud, drawing the attention of the native pedicurist who smiled politely at the English she did not understand. "Gosh, I hope he doesn't quit the project," she added as she jerked her right foot a bit, startling the Frenchwoman. "This could really frustrate Hobby, especially after Cordell and I have approved all of his detailed renderings as final."

However, the truth dawned upon Rachel; she realized that the architect could and would justify countless additional billable hours of design work for implementing her revised, fresh ideas. And, of course, her husband could and would easily oblige with payment. The money spent was of no concern to her. "Anyway, most architects would be thrilled to have the additional work," she added, while jerking her left foot as if to stamp in frustration.

A barrage of *"Madame, ne bougev pas, s'il vous plait!"* was provoked, as the pedicurist practically took off the client's fifth toe as a result of Rachel's unexpected movement. Deep in contemplation, Rachel merely stared blankly back at her, unaware of the near miss.

As her midbrain sensed that Dencil's sense of perfection might not easily embrace her new image for their home, she gently kicked a pile of suds that had collected in a corner of the basin's swirling water surface, the fragrance of the soaking solution made even more overpowering. "Screw Hobby Dencil," she said softly to herself with nervous defiance, but still loud enough for the perplexed salon technician to hear.

But it was her ... their home, she thought further, remaining silent and trying to keep still. The architect would simply have to swallow his own pristine pride somehow and make the changes. He would just have to understand like Cordell was going to; she was totally enamored of the way this rich, heavy stuff looked in the pictorial displays. The catalogue even illustrated where the sections of antique materials had rested in the historic French castle before it was razed, making it easy to envision them in her own castle. Cordell would see it. Hobby Dencil had better see it, too, she decided, kicking reflexively at another mountain of foam. The sudden movement was followed by the seasoned pedicurist's grabbing the leg with a free hand to hold Rachel still as she continued to clip with the other.

"Screw Hobby Dencil!" Rachel declared loudly enough for the next customer to hear as the salon employee finished massaging and drying her American client's toes and feet with a plush, scented towel. Although the woman spoke no English, some words were indeed universal, and she grinned at Rachel, wondering what the American was contemplating. Reaching into her handbag for the tip, Rachel lectured the grinning cosmetologist, "That Hobby Dencil is just going to have to get with the program ... my program ... our program."

Cordell would back her up on this. She knew he would, and she would make it worthwhile to him when he did. With the additional imported materials and architectural fees, the revisions were sure to be expensive, yet Rachel had never sensed any concern from her husband over a shortage of money for their planned home. Throughout their marriage there had been no end to a steady stream of cash, those feelings of financial satiety reinforced by clandestine peeks at any bank or brokerage account statements that happened to surface in her husband's mail at home. Rachel knew what funded those checking balances and investment funds. Cordell or one of his underlings was forever successfully suing people and businesses as those enormous jury verdicts escalated the net worth of Cordell Pixler, a balance he now shared out of necessity with her.

Yes, if she could believe Cordell, which was easy enough, there were plenty of resources to pay for the house construction. Once her husband had purchased a property, he handed all the details over to her, with no budget ever mentioned, and certainly none now.

Oh, my God, it'll look like a 14,000 square foot Taco Bell." Dencil's comment was not entirely a surprise. Once the Pixlers returned from Europe, Rachel scheduled what she termed an emergency meeting with the architect. Somewhere over the Atlantic, a rehearsed Rachel had sketched a totally redesigned front elevation for the Pixler mansion that resembled pictures of that wonderful French castle before its demolition. Her task was reasonably simple since she once again referred to the stolen magazine, this time spread out for reference in the jet's spacious business class section.

"These materials ... these materials ... they're not in union with the concepts we discussed," the inflamed Dencil struggled to say without raising his voice as Rachel presented him with her crude sketches and the catalogue of architectural remnants from River Seine Salvage. He looked over toward Cordell, who appeared as disinterested as anyone who wished to be somewhere else. Cordell Pixler simply wanted his young wife to be content with their new house, content enough to keep him happy.

"But, Hobby, these stones, these carvings, they're all tugging at me. They give me a rush, a rush of history." Almost as an afterthought, Rachel decided to pull her husband back into the discussion. "Cordell and I want our home to be a merger of our spirits. Don't we, Dear?" she asked, reaching for Pixler under the meeting table. As she placed her left hand lovingly on his thigh, Cordell did not flinch, not yet.

"Rachel, this stuff ... these objects ... there's no way to make them functional in the preliminary design of the house, the design you and Cordell have already approved. Nothing about these ... materials ... (Hobby could think of no other gentlemanly term of reference for the architectural pieces that Rachel wanted to use to destroy his design, especially a term that could be used in mixed company) ... even blend with a Georgian style. I have already prepared all these watercolor renderings and mockups for your beautiful house that will fit wonderfully on that gorgeous, established piece of property in Manor Heights. What you're wanting now will look out of place in the neighborhood because it's such a fine, traditional section of Larkspur," Dencil said decisively, pushing his point to the extreme. "In fact, I cannot imagine any place where something like this would fit in," he squeezed out as he pointed to the diagram she had drafted. Hobby Dencil had successfully overcome the indignation in his voice while driving home this point, a quaver more typical of a parent trying to reason with an obstinate teenager.

Without flinching, Rachel stared at Hobby while Cordell only adjusted an iPod he had brought along. Hobby Dencil was just old-fashioned, she believed, his opinionated mind much older than its chronological age. She would not have selected him as an architect if he had not been the most talented of the local or regional ones still accepting new clients. Feeling that her husband's net worth gave her the upper hand, she marched on, "Hobby, I know you can make this work. You just don't want to." Rachel was almost surprised at her persistent, argumentative courage.

Hobby Dencil wanted out of this horrendous scenario. Had he not felt so dizzy and nauseated, he would have believed the entire encounter to be a bad dream, truly more like an endless nightmare. Finding no support from Mister Money Bags still sitting in the leather side chair, scrolling through the iPod, Dencil struggled, "Rachel, I don't design castles. I know I'm responsible for some mighty big houses around the South that some have jokingly referred to as castles, but this concept you have here won't work." He paused for a few seconds, hoping that the foolish woman would regain some sense. "For heaven's sake, Rachel, I'd have to start completely over with the house plans!" he summarized. The break in his speech pattern had elevated to something shy of a flagrant falsetto.

Rachel resumed a debate that she planned to win. Maintaining a fixed stare at Dencil while moving her hand slowly under the table toward her husband's groin, she continued, "We want not just a beautifully exquisite estate but a place where we can raise a family with distinction." She then glanced lovingly toward Cordell, removing her hypnotic stare from Hobby as she pressed against her husband. "I – I mean – we want something unique, something that has not been seen anywhere around here."

Again Dencil pleaded in vain with Cordell Pixler via a useless silent stare directed across the table, an intense look that could never have overridden Rachel's sexually persuasive touch. *"Are you insane? DO SOMETHING. This bitch is creating a gaudy mess that you are going to have to pay for, and you'll never be able to sell it! You must be a freakin' idiot!"* his instincts shouted. As Cordell looked away as though to block transmission of the architect's frantic mental message, Hobby realized that the issue was hopeless. Oblivious to what was transpiring under his office table, Dencil assumed that the moneybags half of this bizarre client package was preoccupied only with an iPod and its earbuds. He believed that such an idiot deserved to be stuck in the monstrosity his wife now demanded.

"Look here, Dencil." The headphones had been removed as Cordell rose to leave, adjusting his pants. "We'll find another architect if we have to. If you're not willing to work with Rachel on this, you can just send me your final bill, and we'll move on to someone else who's less inflexible, some other architect who's less... "

Rachel interrupted before her husband could finish with *pompous*. "Hobby, this French design is what I want. Please work with us." As expected, Dencil then acquiesced after the threats to find another architect, namely his chief competitor in Baton Rouge. He was always a sucker for that argument. After all, it was either shred the existing plans or forgo the cash.

Three weeks later, architect Hobby Dencil and his underling associates and draftsmen had produced an entirely revised set of elevations for the Pixler mansion, spitefully adding another four thousand square feet. The firm's previous design set had succumbed to the office shredder, but not without a few choice profanities blasted by Dencil himself as he personally decimated the discarded plans. Then as he drew out each new room or expanded structural space, Dencil maintained his sanity by tabulating the design hours and ballooning commission that would accompany the revised construction costs. By damn, if the Pixlers wanted an atrocity, he was going to oblige with a colossal one. His reputation could withstand it.

"Jorge, stick it in right here." The classic, trademark *Hobby Dencil Architectural Design* was more than a sign; it was more like a miniature billboard. Typically a point of pride for Dencil, it was crafted of heavy, bold letters – non-tarnishable, tasteful, but distinctive figures – mounted on a faux-metal surface, usually announcing his stamp of approval on the property owners themselves, as well as the project. However, that day as his assistant erected the marker at the base of the Architzel-Pixler property, the sign was a charade and Dencil wanted to kick himself for it. That particular expensive marker was not one of pride in this case, but instead a sign of his overwhelming disdain for the Pixlers.

DARDEN NORTH, MD
200

Chapter

13

◆◆◆

THE GAME

The job would be simple, a rural area surrounded by nothing.

The problem the McDougals faced was shared by many owning real estate unwanted by others — a slow market among certain priced properties, particularly those located in less than popular areas. For obvious reasons, their section of rural northern Mississippi had never been wrapped up in a real estate boom. The land produced only an occasional farming profit, had never been home to once-living fossil fuels, and was too far from a moving body of water to qualify for casino development. But the property was paid for, having been home to a McDougal for as long as could be traced in the family Bible. Except for the equity of sentimentality, the site was of little value to anyone except Mr. and Mrs. McDougal.

Their two hundred-acre farm was adorned with an aging, homely house that had suffered so many add-ons that no one could call them improvements, much less recognize the original structure or floor plan. Despite the couple's growing dissatisfaction with the dwelling, they wanted to hold onto the varied terrain of the farm, hoping for better years ahead for cotton and soybeans.

The problem was the house, the unwanted house.

Both husband and wife shared the domestic dream of upgrading and expanding their living quarters. Initially, they had considered selling the house and building elsewhere on their acreage, tempting potential buyers by including a small portion of the surrounding land in the asking price for the house itself. At least that had been the advice of Darla Bender when the McDougals had listed the property with her real estate firm two years earlier. Bender generally never turned down a client; no prospective sale was too difficult or too insignificant.

Feeling confident that Bender would succeed on their behalf where other agents through the years had failed, the McDougals scoured their land at the time, hoping to locate another site suitable for new construction. The search was fruitless. Not vast enough to be termed *a plantation*, no other area of their property had the elevation, surrounding view, or accessibility of their present homesite. Common sense would explain why. The earlier McDougals had already determined the existing housing location to be ideal. Besides, building anywhere else on the two hundred acres would require installation of utilities.

Two more years had passed, and they were still stuck in what they considered a private dump, an assessment believed shared by everyone searching for real estate in the southeastern United States. Frustrated, Mr. and Mrs. McDougal had been unsuccessful in selling the house even when offering the entire surrounding property for sale. McDougal denounced his wife's alternative of razing the old structure and rebuilding in the same desirable spot since they would forfeit any absolute value of the dwelling. Furthermore, he dismissed as 'too much hassle' the idea of moving the house off and donating it to charity.

Wrapped in marital discord over their housing dilemma and concerned that they would never have a new house, the couple scheduled a meeting with their Larkspur real estate agent. After all, their dead-end selling agreement with Bender had rolled over into its third year, but Darla was about the best real estate agent around. Anyway, they liked and trusted her.

"My staff and I have been working 24-7 on your property. Yes, really pushing it hard over the last ... ," Bender's stretched memory failed her as she smoothly and quickly flipped through the McDougal file lying open before her on the desk. After she located the date of the original listing, she hesitated clumsily and continued, " ... pushing it hard over the last twenty-six months." Her voice faded with embarrassment over the number of months as she winced at the clients sitting in comfortable chairs across from her office desk.

"The wife and I really like working with you, Miz Bender, but we're gettin' a little, I guess you would say, discouraged," responded Mr. McDougal.

"Oh, like I've said before: both of you are dear friends; please call me *Darla*." Darla Bender was as exotic in appearance as her name: tall, almost six feet, but still with a shapely body; long, jet black hair always cut evenly with every strand colored the same dark shade; bird-thin legs to complement her impractically manicured nails; trademark diamond and gold-looped earrings threaded through earlobes that supported pierced diamond studs in the upper cartilage, her tight face wrinkle-free.

"Well, Darla, we've got to do something with this house," McDougal continued. "I guess we should just light a match to it!" he laughed as the missus snickered halfheartedly and continued brooding over the stalemate.

Bender looked up from the short stack of papers on her glasstop desk and stared intensely at the mister, as though reading his mind. She reached into a drawer and withdrew a plain paper notepad, one void of the frilly real estate logo so reminiscent of her other business stationery. Across the top of the first sheet she wrote a cell phone number in block letters. Below the number she wrote *Wayne*. Handing the inscription to Mr. McDougal, she almost purred, "Here, call this number, but use a pay phone. This fellow will be glad to help you. He's really quite good and very thorough."

McDougal looked curiously at Darla as he took the piece of paper, wrinkling his forehead as he studied the note and said nothing.

"Just be sure to call him from a pay phone and pay him in cash. But don't mention my name," she intoned emphatically.

The McDougals never personally met Wayne Simmons. They decided that only the mister would go into the Larkspur Wal-Mart to use the payphone. Lots of people went to Wal-Mart, and he frequently noticed customers using the payphones there, even though cellular usage had become commonplace. She would stay in the parked car, waiting in the lot by the shopping cart corral. Mr. McDougal was sure that his image would be picked up by hidden surveillance cameras because the large store was bound to have them everywhere. He thought about all those investigative television news shows where the police solve crimes by reviewing surveillance tapes at discount stores, malls, and ATMs.

Despite his concern, he decided that this was a good, safe plan since he was just one of a horde of shoppers there that night in the store. Though he felt more comfortable meshing with the crowd of entering and exiting customers around the phone bank, he still found himself fumbling with the receiver and dial pad. Bernie McDougal suddenly became afraid that the old man positioned nearby, checking merchandise and sales receipts of departing customers, would take notice of him or overhear his phone conversation.

McDougal was not exactly sure of what to say during his one and only call to the phone number Darla had provided, so he winged it. "Uhhh, this is Bernie McDougal." As though he had just voluntarily checked himself into Parchman State Penitentiary, Bernie suffered a sudden sinking spell, realizing that he had divulged his name to this Wayne. Maybe he should hang up and just forget the whole thing, he assumed, but then immediately was reminded of his wife's unhappiness. As of late, her daily sulking over their non-salable house had continued into the evening, transforming their bedroom into a morgue. For the sake of those plummeting marital relations, he followed through with the plan.

"First, all I need is an address," said the male voice that Bernie assumed belonged to Wayne.

"Uhhhh ... "

"Hey, look, fella, I ain't got all day. Just gimme the address."

"Route 6, Old Montclair Road."

"Town? State?"

"Oh, yeah. Here in Larkspur. Larkspur, Mississippi."

"Okay, then a rural location. That's easier. Wood or brick? And how big?"

Bernie thought again that maybe he should go ahead and hang up – maybe call another real estate agent or just go ahead and get a divorce. *No, I've got to go through with this.* "Mostly wood, cedar shake siding, with thin orange brick columns supporting the front porch. About 1800 square feet, and pretty ugly. My wife hates it, and nobody'll buy it. The shingles on the roof are curled really bad. We've tried to ... "

"Like I said, guy, spare me the details," Wayne interrupted curtly. "Is there a mailbox out front?"

"Yeah, there's one on the road, right by the gravel driveway. Says *McDougal* on it." As Bernie divulged his name once again, he could hear the door to his jail cell slam shut, and he felt even sicker.

"Who all lives in the house, and what about neighbors? Does anyone live across the street or next door?"

"It's just me and my wife there. We own about two hundred acres on our side of the road, and there are no neighbors anywhere close. Now, there is this abandoned single wide up the road about a half mile. But no one's lived there for three or four years – already covered with kudzu."

"Do you and your wife go out much on Friday or Saturday night?"

"Well, we go to the show sometimes in Larkspur on Saturday, or if there's nothing on around here we'll drive over to Montclair. It's not that far away and anyway there's a Golden Corral right next to the theater."

"Good. Then next Saturday you and the missus leave your house at 6 p.m. Lock all the doors and windows real tight. If you usually leave a few lights on, go ahead and do that. Make it look real typical for when you go out at night."

"Typical, yeah, I see what you're gettin' at." Bernie McDougal was beginning to feel more comfortable with this.

"But this time a few things will be different. Seal $1500 and a key to your back door in a brown envelope and leave it in your mailbox."

"One thousand five hundred dollars?" At that moment, a recorded voice interrupted the conversation demanding more coins to continue the call, startling Bernie McDougal into panicky guilt as though his clandestine activities had just been thrown out into the open and he had blown his parole from Parchman. Gulping to prevent a shriek, he dug into his right jeans pocket and produced enough quarters, dimes, and nickels to satisfy the phone company's minimum.

"Yes, you heard me right. Fifteen hundred, cash. And all must be in small bills, nothing bigger than a fifty. I suggest that you and your wife get the money together separately and do it in stages, you know, a little bit here and there. You don't want leave a lot of paper trail."

Bernie's mind was racing. Fifteen hundred dollars! Was that a lot to pay an arsonist, or was that the going rate? Who wouldya ask, anyway? You certainly wouldn't look it up on the internet. How could he raise that money without creating suspicion? He knew that cashing such a sizeable check or going to the ATM several times in a row would definitely be out of character for the McDougals.

"Oh, and another thing," Wayne's voice added. "No one's going to know who I am. No one will see me, not even you."

McDougal listened intently, all the while wondering if that dinky black dome mounted to the ceiling in the Wal-Mart entrance foyer was recording every move he made, or worse yet, every word he spoke.

"Pay attention, real close now. Here's a little friendly advice," Wayne stressed, but still in hushed tones. He was actually enjoying this call, toying with what anyone would have realized was a highly anxious new client. "You better be sure that you or nobody in your family, and no friends, just plain nobody, is anywhere around your property. Follow the plan exactly like I've laid it out. And don't dare tell nobody where you're going that night or where you'll be."

"Yeah, I see. Got it. *Don't tell nobody.*"

"But the way I see it," Wayne continued, "when they ask you about it later, you was going to the show just like any ol' sweet married couple ... and then out to eat afterwards. Yeah, that sounds like you and the wife was just doin' a real normal thing. Something you do a lot in your spare time, like average Americans.

"Of course, don't move nothin' out of the house beforehand. Leave your things like usual when you go somewhere for a short while. Those fire insurance companies, they'll examine your house with a fine tooth comb. And if stuff is missing, well ... you'll be up shit creek. Remember, don't take nothing valuable with you, except your everyday jewelry and clothes. If you got all that crap inside your house insured, then you ain't got nothing to worry about."

"Yeah, okay. I understand," Bernie McDougal responded even more nervously as the phone company voice warned again of time running out.

Before Wayne ended the call, he added, "I'm going to do you a good job, a real clean one. So if it gets screwed up, then it's yours or the wife's fault. The fire investigator will know where you are, but he'll never find me."

Bernie swallowed hard, regretting that out of this deal he would lose his grandmother's oak dining room table and his favorite hunting rifle. Trying to hold the receiver steady along with his lips, he responded, "Yeah, yeah, that makes sense. I get it. We'll leave the house like everything's business as usual. Just a night out on the town."

"And, fella, when I get to your house on Saturday, I'll first check the mailbox for the money. If it's not there, I'll be real pissed off because you've done wasted my time. And nobody wastes my time and nobody wants to piss me off. After all, I know where you live."

The pay phone went dead, as dead as Bernie McDougal felt at that very moment.

From behind a pile of decaying brush directly across the road, he watched them leave promptly at six o'clock, exactly as instructed, the couple stopping to put a package in the mailbox before pulling completely out of the driveway. After searching their pockets, purses, and bedroom drawers, Bernie and his wife had scraped up about two hundred bucks, the balance pulled from his upcoming paycheck deposit. The McDougals had made reservations at a

Florida motel for the next week to explain the reason for needing the money, should anyone ask.

Wayne remembered the McDougal name long enough to find the mailbox in front of the target, which was indeed located in the middle of nowhere. The modest house appeared exactly as the quirky-sounding guy had nervously described: predominantly combustible exterior, no neighbors. A quick but thorough count totaled $1500, wrapped casually in rubber bands, not bank wrappers, and packed nicely with a door key inside a clean brown envelope. "Good work, fella, just as instructed," Wayne smiled as he put the money inside a vertical pocket on the right leg of his camouflage jeans. The arsonist preferred sand-colored patterns for his professional attire, similar to the military fatigues worn by United States troops in the Middle East. The design coordinated nicely with the tan-colored, surgical gloves he donned before each job. The whole ensemble served well as a standard uniform, whether working inside or out.

The key the McDougals left slid nicely into the backdoor lock. Upon entering the house, Wayne heard no animal noises, particularly no barking, the pet issue being something he had failed to discuss with this new client. He first scanned the kitchen and utility room located to the right, again noting no sign of pets, especially no empty food bowls left at the foot of the refrigerator or near the washer/dryer combo. A dead giveaway for an arson investigator is the discovery of homeowners having rescued their pets even before a fire begins; happily, Wayne found no evidence of such.

"This dude must be smarter than he sounded on the phone," Wayne said under his breath with relief. Of course, he knew that there could be an aquarium somewhere in the back of the house, but he doubted that the whatever-their-names-were would have gone to the trouble to save the fish. So far, Simmons was pleased with himself for taking on this job, one that was lining up to be a problem for his fire investigator nemesis. Wayne believed that all examiners relish exposing fraudulent property cases, especially those involving private homes including lots of unpaid personal property, and Wayne wanted to keep them frustrated.

Many fires that occur in private homes are set by amateurs, the owners themselves. Not surprisingly, their goal is to cash out quickly by destroying the property in an elaborate, rapidly-spreading blaze. From ignorance and unrestricted setup time, the do-it-yourselfers configure multiple points of origin, thinking they are disguising an intentional fire – stupid, convoluted methods immediately obvious as arson to fire inspectors. Wayne despised those amateurs, self-styled arsonists who tried to save a buck to make a buck, instead of engaging a professional like him.

Well-trained in the sleuthlike defensive measures of an expert, Wayne understood that the examiners would be searching the site afterward, hoping for that kind of evidence in this particular case, but eventually come up empty-handed. After all, this was going to be a Simmons fire. Total property destruction that appeared accidental was the signature of Wayne Simmons, his source of increasing personal pride.

Simmons kept his jobs simple, banking on human carelessness and ignorance. An astute businessman, he had correctly assumed a straightforward job when talking to this McDougal, and now that he was inside the couple's home, Simmons congratulated himself. Once again he felt proud satisfaction in his ability to size up the depth and scope of a project with scant information derived from a single telephone call. When accepting cases his ask-few-questions/tell-no-tales policy had backfired only once when he learned later that human remains were uncovered in the rubble of one of his fires. Monetary gain was generally assumed to be a client goal, and Wayne resisted projects bent on human harm.

As Simmons surveyed the site of this commission, he stepped into the living room to find a gold mine. The furnishings there consisted of two foam-padded upholstered couches along with an inexpensive recliner and two smaller upholstered chairs, both with similar foam padding. With his gloved hands he methodically tested all of these pieces by pushing down on the padding. "This junk will make great fuel packages. I just gotta find somethin' to touch 'em off."

Walking quickly back toward the kitchen, he spotted the ideal ignition source for this venture, one that would never be a red flag during an investigation. Sitting nonchalantly on the kitchen counter of this American home was a coffee maker, nearly empty. There were no lights activated on the machine; it was turned off. "Not a problem. I'll just turn it on."

Knowing that homeowners commonly rush out of their houses or apartments leaving such small appliances as coffee makers activated, he immediately decided on his source for this fire. Once the correct temperature was reached, Wayne knew that the plastic section of the coffee maker canister above the liquid would burn vigorously, dropping and spewing plastic droppings everywhere. The remaining coffee dregs would not be of sufficient amount to hinder the combustion. The ignition source now selected, he needed an accelerant – one common to a common home like this one.

"I might want to hire these people as assistants," Wayne laughed to himself as he spotted the week's newspapers piled nearby on the kitchen counter. "They couldn't have made this baby any easier. Maybe I should've charged 'em only a grand." Pushed slightly closer to the coffee maker, the newspapers would be willing fodder for the flaming plastic tossed by the appliance.

Mrs. McDougal's kitchen curtains of simple cotton fabric covering the window above the sink would be the next target for a spreading fire, followed by the paper towels stacked closeby on some open shelving. Banking on his pyrogenic forte, Wayne was positive that in no more than seven minutes of being exposed to an open flame, the room would be brought to flashover condition.

Masterfully, he withdrew a screwdriver from the pouch worn over his shoulders as an undersized backpack and constructed of matching sand-colored camouflage. As able as a skillful heart surgeon performing a long-awaited transplant, he gently picked up the body of the coffee maker and slightly loosened the screws holding the electrical supply cord in place. The objective of this maneuver was to produce an electrical arc, leading toward the chemical oxidation and heat required to begin the flashover.

Maintaining a mental diagram of his methodical fire ignition plan and its pathway of spread, Simmons moved quickly. Next he used the surgical tool to adjust the machine's thermostat and override the manufacturer's safety design. As a result, the heating element would work undeterred, increasing the temperature of the brewing canister to the level of a true melting pot. Finished with the coffee machine adjustments, Wayne gingerly replaced the rear panel to the appliance and smiled with satisfaction. He had used this ignition source on previous jobs, always with a positive result.

Indeed, the trademark of a Wayne Simmons fire was that it was thoroughly executed, even guaranteed. For assurance that the blaze would be a big one, Wayne produced a six-inch, colorfully-decorated rectangular box from his backpack, his trick in this case to yielding rapid combustion and spread. He preferred the unscented brand and often wished he could order the stuff wholesale from the manufacturer, but that would point too many fingers. Instead he bought them at discount stores by the case when available, always careful to avoid surveillance cameras. Before flipping the on switch to the coffee maker, he popped open the box and pulled out handfuls of the fabric softener sheets.

Intended for a domestic clothes dryer, he diverted their purpose by placing the thin paper-style sheets between the coffee machine canister and the base that contained the heating element.

"Burn up, my babies, and then disappear like you always do, without a trace. Yep, you'll make Daddy a nice little explosive flame." In addition to placing multiple segments of fabric softener sheets in and around the coffee maker, Simmons also stuffed several within the pages of the adjacent newspapers and then directed a trail to the curtains where the simple household product would leave no residue after combustion.

He paused for a few moments in the kitchen as the fire began, watching with satisfaction as it spread rapidly. As designed, the flames jumped through the thin ceiling to the attic where the fire would leap throughout the house.

"I hope those people are smart enough to answer 'yes' if some noisy S.O.B. asks about their damned coffee pot – like if maybe they could have left it on before going to the movies?" Wayne summarized while shaking his head. People sure could be ignoramuses!

Certain of yet another successful job, Wayne Simmons slipped back through the door to the outside, blending into the cornfield behind the house to leave a fiery spectacle for no one but him to admire. As he slid into the surrounding darkness, he noticed a backyard propane gas tank, located dangerously near the home.

"I really should have charged these dumbbells less," he decided.

Like any other rookie, I was assigned to the night shift, but discarded as unlikely the thought that Fire Marshal Lisenbe had diabolically stuck me there to keep me from his daughter. Somehow I kept the romance with Kaylee alive during afternoon visits with her in the library after I had slept off my shift. Of course, there were other arbitrarily-timed dates with her.

Despite the bunks provided at the Larkspur Fire Station, we were actually expected to sleep on our time off. There was nothing written about that dimension of the job – it was just understood. A lot of Texas Hold 'Em was played and a lot of television watched during those long evenings of waiting for a building or house alarm to go off somewhere, or a car or truck to collide in flames. Occasionally when we tired of cards, we night owls would collectively rent and watch a DVD.

I had been employed with the department for about a week when our first call to a real fire was received – a real fire, not like the summons during my first night on duty when a skeleton crew attended a three-vehicle wreck on busy Highway 94. Fortunately, no one was injured, and there turned out to be no fire.

However, this call was the real thing, what the new recruits had been trained to handle. By the time we reached that scene on a rural road well outside the Larkspur city limits, it was around 10 p.m., and the house was pretty much gone. There were no adjacent residences or businesses to be endangered, or any one around to care about the destruction except the person who reported the blaze. Had it not been for that adventuresome landowner from several miles away who decided to take a nighttime horseback ride, the Larkspur Fire Department would have remained unaware of the isolated fire that had burned recklessly.

What the interested equestrian first noticed as a curious orange glow in the night sky was deemed a four-truck event by our fire department staff, a sign of the past weeks' level of boredom. Riding the lead truck and preparing to be one of the first to arrive, I silently reviewed the step-by-step protocol of firefighting as well as the proper investigation that accompanies a job done safely. Nevertheless, despite the shrill noise and jerky ride, my mental logarithms seemed to be in place, indicating that Alvin Coakley, my colorful instructor at the fire academy, had taught me well.

Still a magnificent country bonfire when we arrived, the crew and I rapidly contained and doused the blaze, which by then had been reduced to charred bricks scattered among a pile of thick embers and twisted iron work.

When the station received the emergency call, a quick computer search of the city and county records identified the property as belonging to a Mr. and Mrs. Bernie N. McDougal. However, the initial impression of those of us in truck number one was that if Bernie and his family had been confined to the house during the true life of the fire, then they would've joined the pile of ashes. A preliminary search of the site fortunately found no evidence of human or animal remains in the debris.

The remnants of a pickup truck rested in the rubble of what was apparently a carport, a nearly unrecognizable ball of black, contorted metal covered by the cinders of fallen ceiling beams and roofing material. We reasoned that the McDougals were either a two vehicle family or had left their home using other transportation. Another assumption was that the carport section of the house had been flattened by the pickup's exploding gasoline tank. As judged by the degree of structural damage in that section, the truck must have been left almost completely filled with fuel to create such a dynamic fire load. Later investigation would research the gasoline capacity of the make and model.

Even though the house was found in such bad shape by the first-arriving company officer, we in the lead department truck were immediate in addressing the basic differential points between an accidental or intentional cause of the fire. Along those lines, Coakley would surely have been proud of our trained actions had he been present to observe. For instance, as we extinguished the fire we observed no evidence suggesting that the house had been ransacked or had an unusual amount of property removed. We salvaged the remnants of the door and window locks for later analysis and decided that there was only one point of origin – the kitchen.

Around eleven the owners returned home to join a scant inquisitive crowd which had gathered during the proceedings. I photographed the onlookers so that we could later compare this group to pictures of audiences taken at other fires, screening for repeat bystanders. Mrs. McDougal jumped from the car screaming and crying while her husband forced nonchalant control and followed her coolly toward the remains of their home.

"To make a long story short, if this fire was incendiary, then the arsonists did a mighty, if you'll excuse my language for just a minute, damn good job," Alvin Coakley summarized after the property loss insurance company contracted him to research formally the cause of the McDougal house fire. When joining us over a card game one night at the fire station, he shared his findings and thoughts about the loss. The majority of the fire department members sitting around the table had been trained by him at some point or other and relished being entertained once again by an outstanding professor. The rousing game of Texas Hold 'Em enhanced the mood.

"Those folks, the McDougals, seemed to be 'purty' normal citizens, didn't seem to owe too much money – had even paid off the mortgage several years ago. I find it a bit curious that they had tried to sell their house awhile back, but there's just no evidence that they had been preparing for this loss, if you know what I mean." Coakley was to the left of the dealer button, so he and the guy to his left that night, one of our female firefighters, placed the small blind while Alvin did not miss a beat of dialogue. "You guys first on the scene did a great job in your report." Those of us in the lead truck looked around at each other proudly, almost with twinkling eyes, as the tag-alongs turned green. The dealer had dealt each player his two hole cards. The group sitting around the master fire instructor now displayed a mixture of poker faces, some restraining jealousy, but not because of their cards.

"Yep, you fellas did the right thing in checking and cataloguing the contents of the family's storage shed out in the backyard – the one protected from the fire because it was detached from the main house and too far away from that propane tank." The player to the left of the big blind matched it, then raised two, and then everyone bet clockwise. The dealer burned the next card before the flop. Three community cards were then placed face-up on our Formica table as Coakley continued, "You guys even took pictures showing that the shed still housed only the usual homeowners' items like a lawn mower, racks, and garden hose. No sign that someone had coincidentally, ya know, just by accident, stuck a jewelry box, photo albums, or an heirloom wedding dress out in the backyard shed for protection. This morning I snooped around town and found no record that the subjects had rented a local storage facility or moving van recently. And from my sifting through the remains, it also looks to me that the house contents were left in place when the owners left for the night. The closet areas appeared chockfull of clothes and possessions and the rooms full of furniture, or what was left of it."

Coakley continued his summation of the McDougal bonfire as the card game continued. "Also there was no sign of forced entry into the main house or other sabotage. No unusual tools left around. You know, there was this other case that I investigated once; I still sort of laugh when I think about it. Yeah, a real hilarious case that I don't think I've told you guys nothing about. It involved a condom."

"A condom?" several of us asked in startled unison as we studied the three community cards – two sevens and an eight – and placed our bets.

"You mean I really never told this story in class down at Storck?" Coakley inquired, relishing the attention of the masses. "Well, it's a good one. You see, this guy had filled a bunch of prophylactics with lighter fluid and gasoline and used them to set his apartment on fire." The dealer burned the next card and dealt the turn: a king. Now with four community cards, there was another round of bets. The next card was burned.

"The dude then stashed the rubbers under the mattress in his bedroom as well as between the cushions on his couch, even under his kitchen table."

After the final burn, here came the river card: an ace. Our old professor was taking in everything laid out in front of him while omitting no detail of his unique story. The final bets were laid.

"When the investigation identified remnants of those multiple rubber items in the charred remains, the young man was confronted with the suspicious evidence. His explanation was that he and his steady had had a wild and kinky night of it at his apartment before he left for work. But the girlfriend failed to corroborate that tale."

We all laughed, thinking about sex on, or under, the kitchen table between the amateur arsonist and his secretive girlfriend, perhaps even placing ourselves at the scene.

I was holding an ace and a king, making a big slick. My buddy to the right was holding an ace and a seven and won the hand with a full house. He was four dollars and seventy-five cents richer.

Shifting the discussion back to the fresh fire at the McDougals, I asked during the shuffle, "All of us from the department who went to the fire that night believe that it started in the kitchen. What do you think?" Coakley studied his next two down; he was dealer that hand.

Surprisingly, Alvin drank nothing during his visit with us but a bottle of water and only after the third offer.

"The fire had to have started in the kitchen," he answered. "The insulation in the attic directly above the stove area was aged, matted, and highly combustible – burned like sawdust. And it looks like the residents had a bunch of magazines and other paper articles stored up there. There were even a couple of deer heads, or so the husband told us. Fire shot straight up to the attic and lit that house like the wick on a firecracker."

"Do you think the whole thing was a setup?" I asked as the cards were flopped, burned, and the river card was revealed in the next game of Texas Hold 'Em.

"Don't think so. The way it mapped out seems harmless enough. For that kind of crap to be kept in a private storage area like an attic isn't all that strange, especially since the homeowners had lived in that location for so many years. You know, they probably had their income tax returns up there and old bills and receipts – stuff kinda like that."

"The hot water heater was close by the kitchen," another guy piped up as he studied his two cards and mentally laid them next to those lying face-up on the smooth table. He had been on the truck with me that night. "It was just around the corner from the kitchen and must've been a large one for that size house, judging from what was left of the tank. Couldn't that have been what started the fire?" he asked nervously while carefully rearranging the two cards he held in his hand, keeping them very private.

"Hope this doesn't sound rude, but I don't think so," Coakley responded expressionless. "I'll put in three."

"Wow! Seventy-five cents. The pressure's on," I said as I matched his bet and raised him another quarter. All of the players stayed in.

"To make a long story short, I have an idear that it was one of the kitchen appliances, probably the coffee maker. Happens all the time."

Coakley made little of us as he won the hand with pocket aces that looked good, with the ace staring at all of us from the center of the table.

The two thousand bucks burned a hole in her pocket for awhile before coming to rest hidden under a planter. Secure in a water-tight plastic bag, the money would never be exposed for seldom did anyone join Officer Sleethe on the patio. In fact, there was hardly ever a visitor to any section of her apartment.

Because police department employees typically do not have a lot of disposable income, she had been afraid to deposit the money in her bank account or make any show of it at all. Fairly new to the police force, she did not want to be fodder for the gossips of Larkspur's citizenry or raise any suspicion among her superiors. Like the population of most small towns, Larkspur was overflowing with talkers, people who had little else to do but discuss the affairs of others – peanut minds with opposite-sized mouths. She was content in that only one other person knew about the money: the man who gave it to her.

As though on patrol, but actually just off-duty, she would occasionally stroll through the fashionable dress shop, the one downtown by the courthouse. During one such afternoon, she mustered the nerve to browse through the store's scant choices in the plus sizes for short girls. The clerk who walked up to her paused and smiled politely but never really offered to help. No use trying to wait on someone dressed in such ill-fitting, unstylish garb, the dress shop clerk thought – or at least that was what Officer Lyric Sleethe surmised.

Lyric had never seen two thousand dollars in cash before, much less held it in her thick hands – not bad for a few hours work. In return for the favor she had demanded small bills, no larger than twenties, and the man complied. For that matter, he never even hesitated. As she smoothly counted out the money upon receipt and then slid it back inside the small manila envelope, she wished that she had quoted a higher fee.

In truth the young policewoman had been relieved to be rid of me. She reconciled to herself that the money was not really a bribe or a payoff since she had been considering my release from jail anyway. From the minute Sleethe pulled Kaylee and me over in the Home Depot parking lot and forced me from my car, she was concerned that the DUI charge would not stick. Lyric Sleethe knew that her grading of my field sobriety test had been a reckless interpretation, bent on failing me from the start. While there were many DUI arrests each night in Larkspur, particularly on the weekends, her few arrests seldom resulted in conviction. Choosing to improve her arrest conviction record during my single apprehension, she pressed on with the charges under the constant pressure exerted by the Larkspur Chief-of-Police: *Get the damn drunks off the road!* The police chief himself had been given a similar, even more direct ultimatum from the mayor, who was responding to the demands and valid concerns of the citizen advocate groups.

Suddenly Officer Sleethe's gamble over convicting me in a judge's DUI court became an unnecessary risk, as her own low conquest statistics seemed much less important. Greedy human nature pushed ethics aside as unscrupulous profit became a surprising prospect for Sleethe and a solution to my ordeal, one in which Lyric would benefit financially and I would go free. The officer would never have admitted to anyone, even to herself, that she had found me to be a tough cookie during the arrest, though her vigilance never seemed to waver during my perceived torture that night. However, she was happy to have a reasonable and profitable excuse to be rid of me and, though illegal, she decided to make a little cash on the side for a look the other way.

In that small but unexpected fortune, Lyric now saw opportunity.

She had noticed the fellow in that dress shop once before, assuming him to be a rather displaced clerk. Tall, thin, dark-skinned, he was well-manicured, a little too perfect. But on that cruise through the store, the one in which she carried the two grand in a small satchel, he seemed to be involved in more than just simple dress selection. Lyric Sleethe, the woman, not the policeman, moved closer to eavesdrop.

"Sugga, this will be fabulous on you. We'll get your hair all situated, get Persefanie to do it. Put it up like this to let the collar show," he demonstrated as he gently pushed the woman's long brunette hair off her shoulders.

"I don't know, Minor. Do you really think this so? I think this suit makes me look fat."

The man shook his head and shoulders practically in a shudder as his eyes bugged. "Just listen to you. You are a scream. A scream!" Without focusing on anyone or anything else in particular, the man next clapped his hands together and quivered his lips as he glanced around the area. There was no one in the store as thin or attractive as the woman with whom he was talking. "You can wear that diamond and emerald pendant, the one that hangs so well on your platinum necklace. That fabulous thing with this outfit will just put the whole piece over the top."

"I guess you're right, but the skirt may be a smidgen too long."

"Persifanie can fix that, too. This linen suit is exactly what I had in mind when I found that beautiful diamond and emerald thing for your husband to present you with last Christmas. I can still see it now: glowing in the estate jewelry case at the Rexford gift shop when it suddenly jumped right out of the case at me." Minor

Leblanc threw his hands symmetrically above his head as though mimicking an explosion. "That was a Christmas to remember, Girl. You must have been mighty good to ol' Santa."

Certain that the couple remained oblivious to her eavesdropping from the opposite side of the clothes cabinet display, Lyric found the interchange entertaining as well as intriguing. "I know that they can't be married," she muttered under her breath. "They're just too different. He must be some kind of personal shopper or something like that."

"Did you say something?"

Startled, Lyric dropped the blouse she was holding firmly against her breast, a noticeably poor fit. "Oh, no, I was just thinking aloud," she responded to the sales clerk who unexpectedly hovered behind her. The clerk reached to the floor for the silk blouse, looked at it briefly, surveyed Sleethe's physique, and then returned the garment to the rack with a shrug.

The man and the woman finished their purchase and then said their goodbyes. Lyric followed the unique man from the store, using all the trailing skills she had absorbed from the police academy. Happily, the trail was short, lasting all the way to the parking lot adjacent to the dress shop. The plainclothes, off-duty officer stood back around the corner and watched the man approach his car, a bright yellow-colored vehicle that Lyric considered a shrunken type of SUV.

Pulling a pad and pen from her shirt pocket, she recorded the man's license plate number and what she remembered of his name. The customer he was assisting had said it. The name sounded unusual and even though the attractive woman had said it more than once, she still did not quite get it all – started with an *M*, she thought.

Lyric strolled back into the dress shop and returned to the same rack. The clerk spotted her again thumbing through a group of separates, none of which would come near fitting her, although Lyric was studying them wistfully. Even though she could not see the same asinine store employee coming toward her, she could sense it. "Oh great, it's that bitch again," she muttered almost loudly enough for the woman to hear.

"Oh, back again?" the woman asked Lyric, who still dressed in her unflatteringly tight street clothes looked just as out of place in the upper end boutique as she would have in police garb. "Would you like to see something more in your size?"

"No, thank you, Miss ... ," Lyric looked over to memorize the clerk's name tag. The title was then imprinted in her brain, as was the woman's face. Attempting to hide the hurt of being put in her place, Sleethe turned and immediately left the women's clothing and accessories store. Perhaps she would see the clerk again, under different circumstances, and on a different playing field.

Back in uniform the next day at police headquarters, Sleethe ran a computer search of license plate numbers, and in a few seconds there it was, the name she needed: *Minor L. Leblanc,* complete with a recognizable photograph, phone number, and address. Before she printed out the information, the immature but conniving policewoman sat in the work cubicle for a few minutes, staring at the computer screen.

The two thousand dollars would be put to extremely good use – her use. And she would save the clothing store bitch for later.

Chapter
14

•••

THE STOP

The file on the McDougal fire was closed and marked *Accidental*.
A second investigator sent from out-of-state by the couple's
home insurance carrier basically rubber-stamped Coakley's
initial causality report. Yes, everyone was happy. The McDougals
got a new house, Darla Bender no longer had frustrated clients,
and Alvin Coakley looked like a hero – a really smart one. The
Larkspur Police Department had other things to worry about,
bigger fish. Almost as an afterthought, the precinct commander
had assigned one Lyric Sleethe to probe the incident. Since there
were no deaths involved and the criminally spotless McDougals
seemed like innocent victims, she accepted the local fire
department's report as well: *Accidental*.

While the fire and police departments were closing those books
and moving forward to the next inevitably unpleasant incidents,
Hobby Dencil was deep into the Pixler project. House plans for
the expansion of the mansion's planned square footage had been
drawn and redrawn in the weeks following the couple's return
from France. The project was fraught with such indecisiveness that
Dencil ran off two replacement draftsmen after his chief draftsman

of sixteen years resigned in aggravation. As soon as the architect would complete a revised working plan for the Pixlers, one that he himself could stomach, either Rachel or Cordell would envision an additional decadent detail for their home. The number of home fireplaces planned fluctuated more than the stock market, as did the size of the pool.

At one of their follow-up meetings, Hobby tried levity as he jokingly accused Rachel of thumbing through home design and decorating magazines simply to come up with new amenities to include. She did not laugh or even appear embarrassed at the question. "Just redraw it," she responded, to repeat her signature answer. "Cordell will cover your fee. He wants it built right the first time, just as I do. Isn't this what you do for a living, anyway?"

Hobby Dencil answered in the affirmative with a vengeance. While keeping a detailed list of his professional service hours, he revised the plans after each meeting with Rachel Pixler. Cordell began to have excuses for not attending; his mind was elsewhere. As actual construction of the ever-expanding Pixler estate began, the meetings relocated to the site itself, labeled with that prestigious Dencil signage. No driver passing by could miss it, augmented with the lucky property owners' names: Mr. and Mrs. Cordell Oliver Pixler, listed just above that of the Dencil firm. Inclusion of the future homeowners on the sign was not a habit of Hobby Dencil, but Rachel had insisted he revise the initial posting.

Before the first Dencil marker was placed on the property, all remnants of the Architzel structure had been removed. Hobby had made sure of it. Every ember, every broken blackened brick, every stone and piece of metal had been scooped away by the construction bulldozers, all procedures under the auspices of an architect whose trademark was obsession with detail. On the other hand, careful attention was focused on preserving any remaining trees and desirable shrubs. It was not Dencil's intention, but that vegetation would serve as the only living monument to the Architzels of Larkspur, other than my aging Dickens.

Early on some mornings before any neighborhood traffic, the architect would walk the acreage almost in tears as the project began to sprout from the ground. The tears were certainly not for Mrs. Architzel, but out of embarrassment over association with such a white elephant. Hobby had indeed come close to resigning from the project on many an occasion, one notable instance being Rachel's incessant use of a cell phone to converse with others during a personal consultation with him. The purpose of that specific encounter was to persuade Mrs. Pixler from insisting on an ornate Roman statue within the entrance foyer, a decorative detail he had not initially opposed until she asked that it be converted into an interior fountain lit in alternating colors. She barely appeared to pay attention to her architect's recommendations at that dismal meeting, but the message to Hobby was clear – her tennis and Bunko plans were more important at the moment than his assertion of appropriate taste.

After he acquiesced and before he telephoned an Atlanta designer to create the repugnant water feature for the Pixler foyer, Dencil first swallowed two Tylenol PMs. When there was no sedative response, he progressed to a Vistaril tablet, and finally relied on five milligrams of Valium to control his tantrum before making the call. His tolerance to the tranquilizing effects of those medications had built slowly throughout the Pixler ordeal. Initially one Valium tablet would slur his speech. But by the time the water fountain was a reality, he could function on two, operating like a medicated prostitute.

The one professional experience Darla Bender shared with Hobby Dencil was that she, too, had spent countless hours with the

Pixlers, mostly with Cordell and even some of the time discussing real estate. Although she and Cordell had kept their affair entirely discreet, Darla still sensed that Rachel felt uncomfortable around her as the threesome had toured properties for sale. There had been no contractual business relationship between Bender and the Pixlers, only a sexual one between Cordell and the woman Rachel simply considered to be their real estate agent. When Cordell learned of the availability of the Architzel property and purchased it without Darla's involvement, Bender curtly terminated her trysts with the male client.

If you don't need me to broker a property deal for you and that airhead you're married to, then you don't need and won't get anything else from me was her departing commentary. It was not that she really needed the money from the sales commission. For Bender it was the principle of the thing, purely from the point of real estate professionalism. What was even a greater surprise to Darla Bender was that Cordell took her at her abrasive words and did not pursue the affair anyway after he found a piece of property of his own accord. After all, from his perspective the objective to locate an impressive homesite had been met and Rachel kept him busy enough sexually.

Darla Bender's interest in the architectural and construction aspects of the Pixler mission proceeded more as a sideline than as a hands-on project. The cutthroat, business dimension of her life was deep-rooted in winning most battles, although she had lost that one with Cordell. Defeat was unpracticed, and Bender found uncertainty moving ahead in face of it. Once the sale between the Architzel estate and Mr. and Mrs. Cordell Pixler had been finalized and all documents a part of public record, Darla studied them with near fascination. For those materials that were inaccessible electronically, she scrutinized the papers on file at the courthouse as though attempting to memorize the data.

From the periphery Bender continued to follow the progress of an ostentatious project that had amazingly escaped her involvement. Frequently driving by the site during construction of the Pixler mansion, she surprised herself with emotions that mounted daily. She was in denial that her hurt feelings spewed more from consuming sexual jealousy than from simple loss of a real estate commission. While searching for a piece of property for Cordell and his youthful wife, she had often pictured herself as replacing Rachel. Those visions arose from a growing emotional attachment to the attorney – emotion a facet of her existence that very seldom overrode her professional persona.

The anger and resentment over being jilted as Pixler's real estate agent would have nixed her return to any emotional relationship with him, much less a physical one, even if he had pursued it after the deal was closed. However, following the termination of their relationship there was never a telephone call, written note, or even an e-mail from Cordell. Rachel's nonchalant voice mail message canceling the couple's next scheduled appointment was the last indirect communication from her former lover. "We won't require your services further, Mrs. Bender. And we won't need to reschedule," was all Rachel recorded. There was no explanation, and no *thank you*.

Had the real estate broker gotten her hands on the Architzel estate first, things might have been different.

Variation of routine was a mental necessity, if not an obsession, for Lyric Sleethe. Every morning brought another day of dread for her. Directed toward police work after scoring relatively high in criminology on a junior college aptitude test, she began to hate her profession, not for the work it required, but for the image she portrayed: an unattractive female in unisex dress. The Larkspur Police Department salary barely covered her apartment rent and personal transportation expenses, and funds for leisure or self-improvement activities did not exist. Consequently, any sense of ethics had been easily squelched when a two-thousand-dollar windfall was more than she could resist.

Although she often thought about the man she had seen there, Lyric did not return to the elitist boutique during the ensuing weeks, carefully avoiding it even when driving on patrol. Nevertheless, uneventful cruising through her assigned section of Larkspur provided a wealth of time to think about Minor Leblanc.

She kept the information about him hidden in a drawer of her bedside table because no one would find it there. Nearly every night she removed the police department printout and studied it. His latest driver's license picture, current home address in nearby Montclair, and personal telephone number, as well as a generous listing of traffic violations, had been read so often that the information was almost memorized. More than once, Sleethe had dialed eight or nine of the digits of his phone number but pressed the cancel button each time.

Lyric Sleethe had no warning that fate would return this Minor Leblanc to her via the destiny of an easily distracted driver whose odometer was in nearly constant motion.

The Cadillac Escalade failed to come to a complete stop, just rolled slowly through the downtown intersection as it turned in the direction of Manorwood Heights. Officer Lyric Sleethe noticed the infraction, a common one for which she could write a dozen citations per week. The car had a LaVadas County license plate and still appeared clean and shiny even though dusk approached.

Judging from the license plate, the driver was probably a resident of neighboring Montclair. The tag number was familiar; it was the same, the one that she had committed to memory.

It was Leblanc.

She could tell that he was busy chatting on a cell phone, using a handheld unit that remained lawful in Mississippi. Assuming that he was talking with that attractive customer from the boutique or perhaps with the haughty salesperson, the policewoman decided to follow him. Over the next several blocks she thought about the two thousand dollars, lying airtight under the patio plant. To someone like this fellow ahead of her, that amount would be pocket change. The few undersized things she fingered in the dress shop would gobble up two grand in no time.

Remaining oblivious to the trailing police cruiser, the vehicle turned the next corner without giving a directional signal. As it straightened into the far right lane of the boulevard, the expensive SUV was draped in revolving blue lights, dramatic in the failing sunlight. Officer Sleethe could hold her intentions back no longer as she activated the squad car's siren.

"Bye!" Minor Leblanc said flippantly as he was jolted out of the conversation into the reality of driving. Recalling his mounting record of traffic violations over the last few years, his heart sank as he slowed and pulled further over to the right, this time flashing his turn signal. *Oh, Jesus. This can't be happening. Not again.* During his most recent appearance in traffic court, the judge had placed him on probation – one more ticket and his license would be suspended. "I've paid all those silly little fines just like they asked me to," he next said aloud to himself while rapping his right palm against the top of the steering wheel. "Why can't they leave me alone? This Cadillac is my world, my whole livelihood. Oh, Jesus! I've got to think of something, some excuse, a good one!" he exclaimed. Opening the door to head toward the patrol car, he muttered, "I'll be extra nice to this patrolman."

Minor Leblanc. That was the name. Still sitting in her cruiser, blue lights flashing, she recalled his moniker even before the results of the license number search bounced back to her. "Sir, return to your vehicle," Officer Sleethe commanded as the driver stepped onto the pavement in her direction. Lyric smiled as Leblanc scampered back into his car, dropping his designer sunglasses that had been suspended from his shirt collar.

In hope of escaping a traffic ticket, Minor had focused all of his mental might toward bluffing through this stop. This time he needed an excuse, a good one, and as quickly as possible before any of his clients drove by. As it traveled back and forth between Montclair and Larkspur, his bright yellow SUV was readily associated with the name *Minor Leblanc* – that is, within certain circles. Therefore, Minor abhorred the embarrassing process of being recognized committing a traffic offense.

How humiliating, he thought once again. Unfortunately, up to that time all of his previous excuses in similar situations had been pitifully feeble, so ineffective that some officers would issue multiple citations just to shut him up. Now those mounting fines and tickets had become problematic. Due to his poor driving record, he knew that he was nearing the inevitability of license suspension.

Fighting beads of sweat on his forehead as he watched the officer approach though his rearview mirror, Minor realized he needed to change his tactics and fast – maybe try a tough guy image. The apologetic *I'm sorry, Officer, sir, but somebody needs this diamond necklace around her neck in a hurry* tale or the *I've got to get to Mrs. So-and-So's house real quick to help her get ready for the ball at the country club* excuse had never worked. However, suddenly he felt a ray of hope that this time would be different, that he could talk the officer down. The sticky part was how.

Minor's optimism swelled when the patrolman's flashlight beam first whisked across his face, then was directed back to illuminate that of the officer. With enthusiastic shock, Leblanc realized that the patrolman was a woman – of sorts.

"Sir, I need to see your driver's license and proof of insurance."

Minor sensed certain terseness in the woman's voice, terse with an element of nervousness. "Okay, Sugga, now put your lips on and we can talk," he responded in wide smile as he rummaged through his wallet and glove compartment, then glanced back up toward her, realizing that she was not even wearing any lips. *Gosh, she needs help*, he thought as he fumbled again through the booklet of documents, producing the insurance certificate to hand over with his vehicle operator's license. As Minor Leblanc handed the material to Sleethe, his eyes were shaking so rapidly with brain activity that their movement was barely detectable and easily overshadowed by the twitching of his lips. Minor was at such a total loss at what to say or do next that he flabbergasted even himself.

Lyric pulled the light off Leblanc's twitching and shaking and examined his license. As she pointed the beam at the laminated card, she held the heavy, dark flashlight as though it were a club. "Mr. Leblanc," she pronounced his name slowly, with false unfamiliarity. "You failed to stop at that stop sign a few blocks back." She redirected the light onto Minor's face, the eyeball twitching much more noticeably now. "And you did not signal at that last turn," she added.

"Well, I meant to, Miss."

"It's Sleethe, Mr. Leblanc, Officer Lyric Sleethe." Lyric began to transfer the information from the violator's license onto the front sheet of her ticket pad, only she applied no pressure with the pen point. "That's two separate traffic violations. Have you had anything to drink tonight, sir? Any alcohol?" she quizzed, a standard question although in this particular case she detected no sign of open alcohol containers in the car and certainly no smell of such.

"Oh, my Jesus, no" Leblanc said with a degree of indignation that he immediately regretted although Lyric had not heard it over her own mental exercise.

"What's all this stuff in your vehicle, sir?" Sleethe asked as she continued the charade of completing the citation. Lyric enjoyed shining her flashlight in a citizen's face at a nighttime traffic stop, illuminating a distraught countenance as its pupils constrict and its brain fires with potential excuses. She then dramatically shot the beam around Leblanc's vehicle. The pricey SUV was overflowing with boxes and shopping bags, each container brimming with items of women's clothing or jewelry, or both.

Interspersed with the hoard of merchandise packed in his car were diminutive, elegantly wrapped packages. Several shoe boxes with foreign-sounding labels filled the seat floors, which supported a rack of hanging clothes some of which were actually expensive-looking men's blazers and suits. Lyric was amazed at all she saw. She thought back on that day in the dress shop, the exclusive boutique, where she was made to feel out-of-place. This nervous fellow before her was unmindful of her then, but now his attention was directed totally upon her.

"All of these things are for my clients," Minor answered defensively, realizing that he lacked proper documentation authorizing his possession of some of the merchandise, much of it taken out on approval under a longstanding gentleman's agreement with many high-end stores. "I am a personal stylist. I shop for my clients," he clarified.

Lyric looked up curiously from the imaginary record she was creating on her ticket pad. She had witnessed this guy at work at that boutique. He must know what he's doing. *Just look at all this*

crap in his car! she thought. *Thousands of dollars work of crap!!*
The coveted two thousand dollars hidden under a plant on her
patio began to burn a hole in its plastic storage bag.

"You shop for your clients? What kind of clients?" she probed.
The question went unheard as Minor was mentally reviewing his
recent history of traffic tickets and citations for moving violations.

While Officer Sleethe's question was not one of total ignorance,
she was only probing for more information. Lyric already knew
things about Minor Leblanc that he would not have cared to share.
Her earlier search through his computerized driving records had
indeed revealed a long dismal driving history, the significance of
which she had not comprehended at the time. But the detailed
police account of his careless motor vehicular operations was
becoming more significant to her the longer she thought about it.

Leblanc sat staring at the windshield as Officer Sleethe looked
up from the blank traffic citation pad and redirected the flashlight
beam across his face. The facial pigment appeared to have
dropped a level toward pale as his expression now resembled
stone. Nightfall was complete, interrupted only by the passing
headlights which guided those free of such an encumbering
situation. Minor Leblanc was jealous of those law-abiding citizens
who could happily snub the police work proceeding on the road's
shoulder. What he did not understand was their concern was not
in recognizing Leblanc or his vehicle but in remaining incognito to
that squad car as they pushed through post-five o'clock traffic.

Sleethe shook the flashlight only a bit, but still enough to
demand Leblanc's attention from his hypnotized state. "Oh, uh,
yes, Officer. What did you say?" Minor smiled largely as though he
was absorbing Officer Lyric Sleethe in a new dimension.

Dissimilar minds often think alike.

"I asked you 'what kind of clients?' " Minor noticed that his
captor had ceased writing and was resurveying the merchandise

scattered on the front and rear seats as well as in the back storage area. He could sense that the flashlight was darting illumination around the area behind him after flooding the space to his immediate right. His mind came alive with possibilities.

"Mostly sincere ladies and a few gentlemen who are discovering their inner beauty or handsome qualities and desire to be at the top of the social and professional ladders – they want to become better looking and better dressed." The beam had returned to Leblanc's face, bouncing back again to Sleethe, so that unobserved he could study her features.

"Where are your lips?"

"Excuse me?"

"Where are your lips?" he repeated with a visual demonstration that bordered on a pucker.

Reflexively the policewoman touched her left fore- and middle-fingers to her mouth then almost as rapidly jerked them away from her face. "Look, Wise Boy, I'm getting ready to do more to you than issue you a ticket," she threatened as she returned the pen to the pad this time with pressure and thought better of her plan. *Go ahead and write him a ticket.*

"I can't talk to you unless you put on some lips." Minor lit the dome light to his Cadillac and reached across to the front passenger seat.

"Hey, what are you doing?"

"Here try this. As best I can tell under the light of your flashlight, this shade should blend nicely with your skin tone." Leblanc had produced a tube of lipstick from a collection stored in a leather makeup bag. "Yes, this one should be just right for you. Go ahead and put it on."

Lyric glanced around the boulevard, dark except for a few street lights. There was now little passer-by traffic. She closed her ticket citation pad and returned it to the sleeve on her belt.

With an element of hesitation, she took the lipstick and applied it clumsily even with the aid of a lighted, hand-held mirror promptly produced by Leblanc.

"There, that's much better. Never write a ticket without your lips on." Minor exchanged the mirror for the officer's flashlight, directing the beam to better illuminate the mirror so that she could inspect her handiwork more closely. "Now, what about your eyebrows?

"What about my eyebrows?" Sleethe responded while gently pushing her lubricated lips together, working in the lipstick as she admired herself in Leblanc's mirror.

"People were born to have two eyebrows." Officer Sleethe moved the range of the mirror up to her forehead, seeing a thick dark line that extended from above one eye to the other. "You need to wax, wax, wax," Minor Leblanc emphasized as Lyric winced at the thought. "Or you could go to one of those hair removal facilities. There used to be a really fabulous plastic surgery center right here in Larkspur. They had this truly wonderful laser machine – could zap that hair right off, really burn it at the root!" Lyric winced even more noticeably as Leblanc clapped his hands together over the steering wheel, not with fist to palm, but in a truly happy clap.

Suddenly Minor felt odd of his situation. Here he had been stopped for an accused traffic violation made worse by driving a vehicle overflowing with expensive personal items. Yet the policewoman had not asked to see any proof of ownership for any of the stuff.

"You said you were some kind of personal shopper?" the female officer asked him.

"Please!" Leblanc's head vibrated from right to left, in more than just a shake or quiver. "I – am – a – personal – stylist." The clarification was lost on Lyric Sleethe. Her mind remained focused on the two thousand dollars hidden on her patio.

"A personal stylist is more than a shopper," he explained in a suppressed stutter of annoyance. He still hoped to talk his way out of a traffic ticket and preserve his driver's license; however, he had no idea how to do it, not to that point. But he had to do something, because ease of transportation was paramount to his livelihood. One more ticket would finish him off; he would be bicycling goodies all over his hometown of Montclair. But the pedaling all the way over to Larkspur would be rough, real rough, and physical exertion was not his style. Taking a taxi all over northern Mississippi would be an option, but too costly and restrictive for his often spur-of-the-moment services. What Minor failed to consider was that most of his clients would gladly have provided him a driver.

"Listen, whatever-you-call-yourself, I've got two grand cash. How much will that buy me?"

Dissimilar minds often do think alike, for that was the opportunity Leblanc needed.

"Officer, uh," he was still holding the flashlight that was heavy enough to be used as a club and shone it on her name badge for a reminder, "Sleethe" (Minor decided then that the first thing he would change about the girl was her last name), "I receive fees for my services by the hour: $150 for the first hour, then $75 for each following hour. Then I receive twenty percent of the things I ... "

"Nope."

"What'd you say?"

"I said, 'Nope.' You won't be charging me nothing. No fee by the hour or twenty percent of nothing."

Minor's head resumed such rapid quivering that the vibration was again undetectable. The beads of sweat on his forehead then coalesced into a full-fledged stream, flowing down to soak the floppy collar of his silk shirt.

"Mr. Leblanc, or should I call you *Minor*? We're going to get to be very good friends. Real good."

Leblanc's eyelids lifted sharply to blend into the upper portion of the socket, eyeballs so white with astonishment that no flashlight was needed to see them.

Lyric Sleethe continued unabashed with her alternative to an on-the-spot confiscation of the fellow's driver's license. "I've got a certain amount of funds at my disposal. You will agree to shop clothes for me at no extra cost and do whatever else needs to be done to make me beautiful. Makeup, hair plucking, exercise tips, whatever."

Minor wondered how much money this chick really had squirreled away. It couldn't be much more than two grand. After all, she was a policeman, a policeperson. His plan had been a simple talk-your-way-out-of-a-ticket, not a project of unfathomable proportions. *How can I help her?* He wondered. *I'm Minor Leblanc, not Jesus!*

"Well, then, you tear up that ticket, and I'll help you," he agreed, his decision erupting from a mouth disjointed from his better sense. Minor directed the flashlight beam down from her face, tracing the contour of her squatty torso. "This first thing we need to do is get you some Spanx to pull in that cellulite, then lose the polyester suit along with those hips."

Chapter
15
◆◆◆
THE TIARA

    Most likely Larkspur has no more funerals than most communities, but at the time it seemed that more than our share revolved around the circumstances of the Foxworth family. This particular funeral was much less elaborate than that of my parents or grandmother but certainly not less well-attended. Many of Charity Ridley's former students strolled by the closed casket to pay their last respects to the deceased teacher, dropping single flower stems on the shimmering silver metal. The gun blast had destroyed much of the grieving mother's face, too much damage for any mortician to fix. The community was indeed sad for her small local family, once composed of two members and now entirely gone.

    Faith Behneman was appointed executor of her sister's estate, or what was left of it. The liquid assets had been depleted by the final expenses and bill collectors. The bad investments and other intangible spending had eaten away the millions of her remaining cash. Charity Ridley's house was the only piece of her malpractice award left.

Conversely, her attorney Cordell Pixler had managed his take
from my dad's trial with much greater prudence, immortalizing
a large part of it years later in the bricks and mortar monument
constructed for his wife. Nevertheless, by the present phase of the
Larkspur construction project, Cordell Pixler had had enough.
After having surprised even himself with his cowardly bending
to Rachel's emotional demands, he had relinquished all rights
of opinion regarding house plan changes. He had endured more
squabbles involving his zealous, sexy wife and Hobby Dencil than
he could bear: arguments about house design, materials, and
features that were more unpleasant than any courtroom battle.

"I'll never dig myself out of this money pit! It has already
drained me of three times more than we originally discussed,
Rachel," Cordell determined in just below a yell during the last
heated discussion when he opted out of the unpleasant, continued
building revisions. Of course, he was bowing out only mentally,
knowing that payment of the mounting bills and fees would
remain his albatross or at least the responsibility of his secretary
who prepared all the checks. Cordell Pixler had lots of money,
not only the millions acquired from the Ridley malpractice case
years before, but also due to the swelling proceeds from other
legal successes since. Except when trying to keep his wife content
and interested in him, Pixler knew how to maintain and grow his
wealth through prudent, though many times ruthless, investments.

While Rachel Pixler may have been content in her husband's
indulgences, Darla Bender had a different take on the construction
of the Pixler Estate or *Pixler Palace,* a moniker coined among real
estate circles. Although the timing was off, she would have had
the perfect property for her former clients, Cordell and Rachel
Pixler. Had they been only a tad bit more patient, she could have
sold them the property recently made vacant by the Ridley suicide.
Moreover, she believed that if the Pixlers had been forthright with

her in their search for real estate, she would have understood their desire to acquire a construction site rather than an existing home. And typical of a top-notch broker, she knew of the perfect construction site – it lay under the crumbling Ridley place. The single recommendation of the house inspector was to scrape the house off the lot and start over.

In bemoaning the lost opportunity to have sold Charity Ridley's house and grounds to the Pixlers, Bender failed to recognize the potential awkwardness of that transaction: Ridley had been a legal client of Cordell Pixler and ultimately a dissatisfied one. But that concern was lost on Darla Bender – a sale was a sale, a commission was a commission. Do whatever it takes.

The Ridley property stalemate now presented a challenge to Darla Bender's rank as one of the top real estate producers in Mississippi, if not in the Southeast within her size market. While Charity Ridley had chosen to end her life outside the house so as not to mar it physically, an emotional stigma enveloped the property instead. The haunting legacy of tragedy – daughter's untimely death followed by mother's fleeting prosperity followed by suicide in the backyard – challenged even the veteran broker, who had smelled a sizable commission when the estate contracted her listing services. Despite the inarguable beauty of the property's grounds, the bloody site near the rose garden long since gone, the skills of Darla Bender had not been able to move the property.

Furthermore, the tragedy surrounding the Ridley family was not the only problem keeping that real estate commission from Bender. Discovery of concealed asbestos under a replacement roof, termites thriving throughout much of the house, and an unstable foundation had spoiled the first sale, initiating a downward spiral of property value and foiled attempts to dump the site. However, clients like the Pixlers would have been the solution. Razing the house and outbuildings for a new high-end structure was the only answer, but that concept was beyond financial reach of most in Larkspur, except the successful attorney and his wife.

Driving by the Pixler project and watching the evidence of a missed sale was more than Darla Bender could tolerate. When she confided her frustration to one of the subordinate sales agents, the response was given with a smirk, "Why don't you just take a different route through Manorwood and avoid it?"

That solution was too amateurish and ended the young man's career with Bender and Associates. The principal's dealings with the Pixlers had been one of her few professional failures, not to mention a devastating personal disappointment.

Bender had exhausted every avenue in trying to satisfy Rachel Pixler before the two finally trumped her. During appointments with Rachel, none of the homes available for sale (even in the newer areas of Larkspur) were ever adequate for the attorney's wife: never large enough, never trendy enough, never in a truly exclusive spot. Therefore, the concept of locating a basically suitable structure in a desirable neighborhood that could be totally remodeled and expanded was first broached by Bender herself. But then Mrs. Pixler decided to carry the concept to the next extreme: find the ugliest or even most beautiful house on a wide, deep lot in Manorwood Heights, buy it, and then just scrape it off. The real estate broker was impressed by the wife's refreshing openness which still bordered on childish. "I'm sick and tired of this BS, Darla. Talk somebody into selling their house, damnit Cordell has sued enough people to afford whatever it takes."

From the moment she had been approached as their real estate broker, it was obvious to Darla that money was of no concern to Mr. and Mrs. Cordell Pixler. Cordell repeatedly reinforced that impression during both business and what would quickly become intimate exchanges with her. His physical and emotional attentions had seemed genuine, a need for real diversion from

the immature, whining, and demanding wife whose amorous
libido would at times dramatically diminish. From his dress and
imperial manner, Darla judged that the legal business must be
good and Cordell, apparently good at it. And from the outset of
their relationship, she had planned for him to spend a substantial
portion of that goodness on her.

However, it was Cordell who profited most from the dealings
with Darla, although indirectly. Darla had kept both of them busy,
brokering more than real estate. For Rachel it was handholding
during time spent searching for a dream home that did not
yet exist. For Cordell it was a physical release temporarily left
unsatisfied by a spoiled, petulant wife still living in the leftover
environs of the previous Mrs. Pixler.

Cordell's undermining of his lover's business efforts ended
their sexual relationship as though that had been his intention all
along. Once he usurped her enterprising and typically successful
brokerage efforts by seizing the Architzel property himself,
Darla had expected, at the very least, an apology, although no
appreciation or expression of regret ever came – just that curt
phone call from the gold digger. Cordell Pixler, Esquire, had done
what he did best: pull strings and tighten ropes within the auspices
of legality, this time to screw Bender Real Estate.

Darla's agony over the whole situation was compounded in that
she could have been recognized as broker for the deal. Ultimately
his overindulged wife would still have been equally as pleased, and
Cordell could have kept Darla and she, him. But maybe he had not
really cared about her. That's what really hurt. Cordell Pixler had
scraped away Darla Bender in one fell swoop in much the same
way his wife could have scraped the Ridley house off its
lot – asbestos, insects, cracked cement pilings and all. Instead
the Ridley house still stood unsold adjacent to the Architzel
ashes, which had succumbed to a bulldozer to make way for the
Pixler Palace.

Regardless, Darla Bender's resentment toward Cordell arose from a double offense: she was both cheated out of a real estate commission and dumped from a fairly satisfying sexual relationship. Her thoughts over the ensuing months had bounced back and forth between the two hurts. Truly, which was worse? After agonizing over that one-sided debate, she determined that forgiveness for Cordell would have been possible only if he had been truthful with her. Instead, Cordell had not been honest. His overriding concern was to keep Rachel Pixler happy at any cost, that deception clear in the final, silent treatment of Darla. While he had assured Bender of his empty, dead-end marriage, the delicate, deceitful whispers had been one long sexual lie. Through all the personal discussions and efforts to locate a new house, the real estate broker had not seen through his false promise that the place he sought would eventually be Rachel's alone.

Those lies now burned deep inside Darla Bender, the hurt surfacing like vomitus each time she drove by the rising Pixler Palace. Initially she had slowed to survey the house and its out parcels in ridicule. But soon she could no longer look at any of the monstrosity, turning her head from the torment while nearly running her vehicle off the street.

Based on another business deal, Bender's mounting disdain for Cordell Pixler was even further fueled. His legal firm had handled the closing purchase transaction of Charity Ridley's home that had eventually shown itself as no more than a crumbling shell. What the house inspector uncovered during Darla Bender's first failed attempt to resell the Ridley estate had gone shamefully undiscovered by Charity's then-trusted advisor, Cordell Pixler, Esquire.

Cordell had done more than merely advise Charity Ridley when she purchased the doomed estate in Manorwood Heights. His firm handled all of the real estate transactions in obtaining the house and grounds for her, again squeezing out brokers like Bender. At the time Darla had accepted Cordell's thin explanation for using his own licensed staff to usurp the real estate transaction. "The poor woman, Mrs. Ridley, and her only sister spotted the listing in the *Larkspur Ledger* while checking out at the grocery store and asked if I would handle the sale. You know, she was comfortable with me and wanted to keep a real estate broker out of it," he detailed. "She was concerned about expenses and extra real estate fees, I guess." The ambiguity of the explanation was that at the time Charity Ridley still possessed millions of her medical liability settlement, millions later burned through scams and unwise investments. Nevertheless, Charity saved nothing by using Cordell's real estate acumen since he pocketed the same brokerage fees that would have been paid to Darla Bender.

Feeling like the consolation prize from that deal, Darla was now saddled with handling resale of the undesirable Ridley home which had sunk to depths of a real estate trade rag displayed among newspaper tabloids. The *Larkspur Ledger* advertising department would not even touch it.

While Darla Bender felt the stinging rejection of the Pixlers, a snub that was both emotional and financial, Faith Behneman was dealing with her own resentment stemming from the dismal state of her late sister's Larkspur house. Initially unsure of where to focus that bitterness, the anger was soon directed at her own disintegrated life and the inheritance she felt had been stolen from her and her children. That bequest which had seemed a grand estate left to her by Charity Ridley was now determined as worthless except for the land on which it stood. Faith Behneman was overcome with angry hopelessness, the kind of resentment that overrides even common sense.

The value of her late sister's house, or the lack thereof, would not have been so paramount had Behneman still retained her own portion of my father's bloodletting. The two daughters' string of beauty pageants had definitely taken their financial toll on the gift check received from Charity, sliced from the final medical liability judgment. Those contests held throughout the state of Mississippi had drained not only Faith's reward for being such a devoted, helpful sister but also had emptied her personal savings.

The enormity of the expense related to the steps of pageant competition was matched only by the degree of disappointment for her two children. Both were left tear-stained and miserably empty-handed when the roses and crowns were handed out; neither was even ranked among the top ten contestants. So sure was Faith that at least her older daughter would win the state crown that she had already begun to piece together the girl's wardrobe for the national contest. Not that Faith felt she could blame her daughter, but the devastated older teenager steadfastly refused to wear the clothes even socially. Once her chances for advancement to the national pageant were gone, the girl swore off beauty and talent contests forever, regardless of the opportunity for college scholarships. The expensive gowns along with the other more casual clothes were left to hang unworn and discarded in her closet. Likewise, Faith's younger daughter took a dismal stance of the future once her junior pageant dreams were also dashed.

By late August of 2005 the dreary Behneman household in Pass Christian, Mississippi, was left without a hint of joviality, all happiness sucked away by the judges' decisions. Faith still found herself unemployed after hastily resigning her longtime job to pursue pageantry fulltime, her fateful decision having been cushioned by the house and cars she had owned outright, along with the sister's check, now completely spent – and then some. In the style typical of resilient teenagers, Faith's girls went on with the start of a new school year, the younger still in high school and the older a freshman at Southern.

Not unlike her daughters, Faith's positive feelings were beginning to resurface as a few job prospects presented themselves. While her previously abandoned accounting position was closed to her, a result of burning too many bridges, promising opportunities had materialized in the business offices of more than one bustling casino illuminating the Mississippi Gulf Coast. Tragically, that optimism was derailed as the largest hurricane ever thought to have landed on the soil of the United States either blew or surged away Faith's improving financial position as well as the lives of more than a thousand people. Joining the casinos and other business structures strewn along U.S. Highway 90 in the aftermath of Hurricane Katrina was the only piece of personal financial security left for Faith – her own house.

The home in which she had raised her two daughters was leveled to a sand-covered slab before a panoramic view of the Gulf of Mexico. All of the Behnemans' possessions, except a few suitcases packed hurriedly for the hurricane evacuation, were sucked into the invading gulf. Once the authorities allowed evacuees to return to the coast for property inspection, Faith Behneman found few remaining landmarks leading to her modest former neighborhood. Gone were the street signs and many of the streets themselves, also buried in sand if not in pieces lying somewhere in the bay with the automobiles, appliances, and the missing persons. As though it had never existed, the familiar convenience store marking the turnoff to her street from Highway 90 had disappeared, probably swept into the gulf when the water's surge receded. Where Faith would have expected her neighbor's brick house to stand, there was nothing left, not even a brick.

But twisted among some leafless oak branches of what remained of her front and backyards, Faith found telltale clues of a devastated family, her family. Glittering remnants of jeweled pageant gowns tightly decorated the treetops of the small acreage,

resembling colorful paper and wire garbage twist ties, strangling
her last hopes and dreams. The waste served as a beacon for an
angry mother, calling her home to yet another disappointment. As
Faith Behneman continued to walk carefully among the stench of
decay emanating from unidentifiable trash and debris, she reached
a familiar ditch that served as the property's boundary. Scattered
among the debris filling the trench were tattered, crinkled
fragments of well-thumbed fashion and celebrity magazines,
manuals for a lifestyle that she no longer considered important.
As Faith continued through her personal aftermath of Hurricane
Katrina, she fell to the sand in tears, engulfed in futility and grief
that was the culmination of the preceding long months. Somehow
the vanity of all her efforts, all of the unachieved goals for her
daughters, pierced her heart as she felt it implode inside her chest.

The tears progressed to wailing heard by no one as she cried
for what seemed like hours. Finally Faith stood, knocked off the
sand and dirt, and continued to stroll in anguish. She found it a
half mile from her homesite, buried under a wheelbarrow in a
pile of other debris and easily recognizable from many feet away.
Jumbled among the contents of a destroyed garage storage room,
the trophy was all that was left of her older daughter's bedroom.
The once coveted prize of a minor, regional beauty pageant, the
rhinestone tiara rested atop a soggy, rotting mound of junk.
No longer was the formation of molded plastic and rhinestones
crowning a hopeful bedroom display of ribbons, certificates,
and eight-by-ten photographs. Instead, the swirling wind had
placed it there to cap a pile inhabited by ditch insects, mold, and
bacteria. But for Behneman, the storm's relocation of the spoils
of pageantry was a deeply penetrating symbol. Now the layers of
rhinestones crowned a mound of loss, a misdirected use of time
and resources, a mountain of mistakes.

Faith reached for the headdress, careful to avoid the rusting nails protruding from a jagged piece of nearby lumber. She immediately envisioned her elder daughter, proudly parading the cheap emblem of victory across a diminutive auditorium stage. As the beautiful daughter displayed impeccable posture, the tiara was supported above streaming tears that marred her expensive facial makeup. Faith had hoped that those Saturday night accolades would result in something more substantial, a weightier crown to follow – heavier not in the sense of physical weight, but in the sense of greater prestige. All those hopes were dashed by those ignorant judges at the state pageant, those tuxedoed assholes sprinkled among a panel of aging, faded beauty queens from another era. During the pageant those queens had smiled so beautifully at the camera during the judges' introductions, and Faith had admired them as gods. Why had those gods been so unjust? Why hadn't they seen her daughter as everyone else saw her: the most gorgeous, the wittiest, and the most talented?

The distraught mother paused with the tiara pulled against her chest and in panoramic fashion gazed at the sickening earthly spectacle before her – upturned vehicles, distorted washing machines, boats perched in tree tops. Those celebrated, jeweled male and female pageant judges were draped in garments surely more costly than the college educations Faith would no longer be able to afford for her daughters. Several years of free college tuition would definitely have eased this unexpected financial burden now surrounding Faith, a financial burden that had engulfed her just as the devastating storm had obliterated the world around her. If only there could have been some pleasant moment in the Behnemans' recent past – if those bitch and bastard judges had just placed her older daughter somewhere in the top five of the state pageant, she would have received a decent scholarship.

"Don't give up. We can learn from your mistakes. We'll take

more lessons, switch coaches. Maybe your little sister'll have a chance," she told her older daughter after her loss in the state pageant.

"What mistakes, Mom? That shitty thing was rigged!" the girl broke into a tantrum at Faith's plans. "Remember one of those damn judges, the made-up blonde, the one that looked like a whore? During my talent and swimsuit preliminaries, I watched her real close from the stage. She never even looked up at me. She probably couldn't since her neck was so tight from plastic surgery. She probably had her freakin' mind made up before the freakin' pageant even started!" she blurted out to her mother, even more hurt by Faith's vague and unintentional criticism than the aftermath of the disappointing decision.

In a burst of anger and frustration, Faith tossed the tiara back into the pile of rubbish with a flick of her wrist. She saw no reason to take it back to the Jackson motel room which had been the Behneman site of evacuation from Hurricane Katrina. The piece would only serve as a sad reminder of her dying, disenfranchised family. Despite its flimsy construction, the headpiece survived the near projectile fall into the shallow ditch, but not the crushing blow of Faith's heel as she climbed down and flattened it.

The hurricane thoroughly removed any semblance of teenage normalcy for the Behneman girls when it erased their private school buildings as well as their home and belongings. The academies and classmates were scattered by the wind and water along with the required prepaid tuition, simply one more financial loss for their despondent single mother.

After returning to sit alone in the Jackson motel room furnished by FEMA, Faith fretted that the government's pecuniary support of her plight would evaporate as quickly as did the value of her sister's home. While Charity's death had been just as heartbreaking and unexpected as the hurricane that eventually followed, inheritance of that property in Larkspur should have been a financial nest egg for Faith – one that she had not planned to need so frantically or so soon.

She now realized that her monetary dependence on that real estate in Larkspur had been as ill-advised as the reliance on her own home's casualty insurance policy. Faith had missed the document's fine print: *property damage secondary to floods not included.* Despite the two-hundred-plus mile per hour winds of Katrina, her home had been washed away, not blown away, or so the insurance adjustor had said. Her local insurance agent, the fellow who had pocketed a healthy percentage of her premium expense through the years, was suddenly absent to address her coverage concerns. As telephone calls to him from the Jackson motel sanctuary went unanswered, she assumed that the agent had either met his own fate or had relocated to a comfortable place where something was left to insure. Almost ashamed of herself, she wished the bastard was pinned under a washing machine, rotting somewhere out in the Gulf of Mexico.

As Faith's anger and frustration over the situation mounted, the insurance company's corporate office continued to deny her appeal of lack of coverage. Each time she called the toll-free telephone number and punched the number 2, then 1 then 4 then 6, and then back to 2, the information related was always the same: *Coverage for flood damage or loss is excluded as itemized under the policy Exclusions Section. Thank you letting us service your insurance needs. Please call back if we may help you further.* Faith followed the voice prompts every time, merely encircling the series of numbers that led to the same disappointing end, which had really been the beginning.

Despite her fruitless attempts to resolve the dismal situation, Faith became the recipient of a string of communiqués, all unsolicited. Amazingly, the letters and phone calls found her despite her uprooted state, originating and drafted by various attorneys from various locations offering to help "ill-fated individuals" like her "during these regrettable times." Even though FEMA was temporarily paying for the single motel room for her and her two children, the agency, citing some technicality, had thus far refused to help with the cleanup or rebuilding of her particular property in Pass Christian, and there had been no promise to rectify the delayed assistance anytime in the near future.

Alone in that motel hovel in Jackson while her younger daughter attended a local public school and the older remained in college in Hattiesburg, Mississippi, Behneman terminated her final frustrating call to the insurance company. Although Faith had paid little attention to it, the television at the front of the room had been on for the last several hours as she lay in the dark, curtained space on Interstate 55. Abruptly her stupor of self-pity was broken by the commercial, the audio of which seemed to project louder and more noticeably than the preceding programming.

The advertisement hawked an adamant lawyer. "We must bring the big insurance companies to justice. Join me in tracking down those unscrupulous insurance agents. Let's make them pay you what you deserve. I can help you. Call our toll free number at the bottom of your ... "

Faith grabbed the remote, snapped the hawker silent, and then threw the thick, black plastic device across the room. It slammed against the television screen, which withstood the impact better than the remote itself, the batteries inside popping lose to hurl against the door with a dual thud. She was disgusted with lawyers, disgusted with the whole legal system for that matter. Behneman faulted herself for not having assisted her late sister in the purchase of that expensive but now worthless house in Manorwood Heights. However, just as she had been confident in her insurance agent, Faith had shared Charity's unflinching trust in the trial lawyer.

"Mr. Pixler promised he would continue to help me. He's going to take care of everything for me. Help me put my life back together." Charity's remarks of self-assurance whirled in Faith's besieged conscience. Her deceased sister had shared the attorney's promise during a cellular chat held shortly after the malpractice judgment was final. However, being a single mom with two busy teenage daughters, Faith held her own personal concerns and had already devoted considerable energy to her sister's plight.

"Let that attorney go ahead and deal with Charity's problems. I don't have anymore time to share," she had said to herself while hurriedly disconnecting the call.

As the final legal proceedings unfolded and were laid to rest, Faith's perception of Mr. Cordell Pixler, Esquire, was clear: the attorney had selfishly pocketed a huge chunk of what the jury had meant for Charity. Faith was sure of it; at least she knew of the jury's intentions. After all, Charity was the one who lost her beloved daughter at the hand of the doctor and his plastic surgical center. No amount of money could have eased her dead sister's mind, although those people in that courtroom, those wonderful people, sensed a mother's agony caused by the torture of incompetence. Those twelve passionate, intelligent individuals on that jury could not bring dear Flowers back, but they had done the only thing possible. They made the doctor pay and made existence a little easier for Charity.

For that reason there was no question in Faith Behneman's mind. What the jury had not intended was not to fatten the coffers of the lawyer, that Cordell Pixler. Yes, Mr. Pixler had indeed dealt with Charity, dealing her a bad hand as he took care of *everything*.

When Charity received her final court documents and financial proceeds, Faith was astounded to learn how much

Pixler had siphoned off her sister's judgment: including expense reimbursement, more than fifty percent was allocated to the attorney's firm. She pulled a cheap calculator from the purse she had tossed on the bed and, as she had done so many times before, punched in the numbers. The thief had pocketed well over half of what those twelve just citizens had intended for her sister. "That bastard! Over fifty percent of my, I mean her, money!" she screamed as the calculator met the same fate as the television remote when another legal services commercial appeared on the screen.

"More lawyers screwing the little people just like doctors do. But that doctor is dead!" Faith shouted in the motel room off Interstate 55 as she slammed the television off at its console control and stormed the short distance from the bed to the sink and dressing area. Absentmindedly, she returned her purse to its usual spot on the open closet shelf above her clothes, losing grip of the handle while looking in the direction of the toilet. The purse, a famous designer knockoff, fell from the shelf, bursting open on the thin all-purpose carpet which covered the concrete slab floor.

There it was, appearing almost prophetically from all the junk once crammed into her leather handbag as it landed appropriately near a miniature, white plastic wastebasket. The brown, letter-sized packet had been missed earlier when Faith shuffled through the mail given her by the motel desk clerk. Stooping to pick up the thin packet, Faith tore it open with a wary degree of anticipation as she noticed the return address.

She read the letter quickly as her heart raced, then met the disappointment of a repetitive, never-ceasing cycle. It was another rejection notice as the federal government continued to let her down. Contacting the National Flood Insurance Program had been a long shot. She knew her property had not been covered by that agency, but for some reason she had expected an element of pity, possibly a miracle. As though in an effort to ease the rejection, the correspondence from the NFIP detailed the dismal financial plight of the service, now bankrupt and of little good to anyone regardless of eligibility. It seemed that other victims of Hurricane Katrina and her younger sister Rita had scored early by submitting their claims before the fund's $3.5 billion was disbursed.

"Those lucky jokers must have had somebody good around to tell them what to do," Faith decided after studying the body of the letter. Yesterday she had read in the Jackson newspaper, *The Clarion-Ledger*, that the NFIP needed more than twenty billion dollars to reimburse the remaining hurricane victims that actually had verifiable flood insurance. The article detailed that Congress had approved a mechanism for the National Flood Insurance Program to fund remaining legitimate loss claims by borrowing money from the United States Treasury.

"Well, hell! That big fat loan won't help me," Faith said as she spotted another letter in the pile of clutter erupted from her fallen purse. Typical of the many others she had received, this one was from a Florida attorney also licensed in Mississippi. His gracious offer was to represent her in a suit against FEMA and other applicable agencies of the United States government for failing to help her with significant financial assistance. "Bloodsuckers, that's what they are. They don't really want to help me; they just want to reclaim my money in my name, then take most of it for themselves," she cursed, using surprising dexterity to rip the correspondence into minuscule pieces.

"I hate those freakin' bloodsucking lawyers." Faith liked the description and repeated the characterization. Somehow hearing the words gave her a sense of satisfaction. "Yeah, even if the asses collected any money for me, they would keep most of it. And get away with it! All nice and legal, just like what that Mr. Cordell Pixler did to me. I mean to Charity."

She ripped the Florida lawyer's letter into even finer pieces, building a neat pyramid on the cheap carpet. An electric paper shredder set to *confetti* could not have done a better job.

Chapter
16
◆◆◆
THE PALACE

Move-in day approached.

Hobby Dencil had considered an escape to Europe like his clients, but the call from his pocketbook beckoned him to stay. During the construction of the Pixler estate, his pride and self-esteem had been destroyed as his money market account escalated. The Pixlers had been prompt with payment and each interchange with the worldly couple was finalized with the same direct nod from Cordell: "Keep her happy."

Dencil picked up on the moniker at a cocktail party in Montclair given by a group of doctors, finding it initially embarrassing but later realizing the humor in it. *The Pixler Palace* reference was whispered to Hobby Dencil in jest during the aftermath of an introduction over Jack Daniels. In fact, he and his draftsman privately used the nickname among themselves, careful not to let it slip into conversations with Cordell or Rachel Pixler.

"Oh, so you're Hobby Dencil. I saw your name on this huge sign in front of a construction site in Larkspur, in my brother's neighborhood," murmured one of the doctors upon introduction to the esteemed architect. "Hell, there was no way to miss it. My wife and I were over there last Saturday for a late lunch and rode around the neighborhood for a while before driving home. We slowed down at the bottom of that hill for a good look at the house. No, it's too big to be called a *house*. I wanted to pull the car up the drive and walk up those steps, but my wife wouldn't let me."

The architect suppressed his embarrassment by mentally reconstructing his latest money market account statement. "I need to shift some of that over into mutual funds," he silently decided as he swallowed the biting liquor, taking a larger sip than planned.

"Yeah, that's quite a place you're building over there in Manorwood Heights. Makes my brother and his wife's place look like shit!" The other men with Dencil laughed softly, knowing that the brother's place was itself a sprawling spectacle.

"Actually, I'm only the architect on the Pixler project. Larkspur Construction Company is handling all of the contracting work. I retain quite a bit of input into the materials and workmanship detail, though, as I do on all of my projects," Hobby responded truthfully but with slight hesitation. He decided that hearing himself admit his continued involvement with the Cordell Pixlers and their monument to financial success had to be as painful as any of the darkest Catholic confessions.

"Yeah, that's quite a palace you're putting together over there," the physician repeated as though Dencil had not just spoken. "Those Pixlers have themselves quite a palace, and I know where it came from. Too bad tort reform hadn't kicked in by then."

"Oh, yeah. That's right," agreed several others grouped around, almost in unison.

Hobby Dencil felt even more uncomfortable in the conversation. He knew that as a plaintiff's lawyer Pixler had first rocketed to financial freedom with a malpractice verdict against some doctor in Larkspur, but he had never questioned the source of any client's income or ability to pay his fees as long as the resources appeared legal.

"Boy, that Pixler. What a scumbag. Sued one of our brethren, my dear fellows. And sued him real good!" The talkative doctor exclaimed to the attentive peer group, now ignoring Dencil and becoming even more gregarious as he neared the bottom of a third glass. "Cordell Pixler made off like a bandit in that malpractice case against Foxworth over in Larkspur. Hell, Foxworth lost his damn practice over it, and all his partners left town. Then Pixler started to build himself a damn palace. Hell, might as well call it the ... yeah, might as well call it the Pixler Palace."

The other men laughed again, this time with much more definition than a mere snicker as Hobby Dencil edged away to return to the bar.

He was behind, way behind.

The hot flashes and night sweats were becoming intolerable. Even a night of cocktails could not muffle his thoughts as he replayed the comments regarding the Pixler Palace. Hobby Dencil had not slept in weeks. During summer visits to his aunt's house, he remembered overhearing her discussing similar symptoms with friends during their cocktail hour on the patio. Only his own lack of sleep was not due to fluctuating hormonal levels associated with that of a menopausal female, but instead was linked to the outrageous ideas of a much younger one.

"Hobby, I just won't have it!"

Dencil hated himself almost as much as he despised Rachel Pixler for her stubborn streak, her near obsession with grandeur. Never before had a client been so overbearing, so persistent – particularly one whose spouse or partner exerted little to no financial restraint. Sometimes the repeating floor pattern of Rachel's proposed Meditation Gallery flashed before him at night in bed, the recurring pattern of diversely shaped wooden pieces stained in various hues almost blinding. As close to a psychedelic trip as any other experience, he would thrash alone in his king-sized bed on those insomniac nights, visions of alternating geometric designs flashing and blinking before him in a myriad of colors as they swallowed him whole.

During one of those long nightmares caused by the antics of Rachel Pixler and spent in drenched, tangled bedclothes, he rammed his fists against the thick mattress. Irritated, his sleeping cat then jumped for other cover under an antique rosewood chest. Grabbing a pair of tennis shoes, the frustrated architect followed the cat's lead but instead headed for his Lamborghini. Hobby's 2 a.m. mission was a last-ditch effort to rework the façade drawings of the Pixler Palace and transform the monstrosity he had been forced to create.

The drive to his temporary downtown Larkspur office was fraught with flashbacks of the many tortured hours he had spent with the Pixlers, mostly meetings alone with Rachel. He could almost see her face in the headlight beams and wished the rest of her would materialize in the vehicle's path.

"What do you call a southern woman with an obsessive-compulsive personality?" a stand-up comic on the XM radio station seemed to ask Hobby personally.

"A bitch," Dencil answered, beating the entertainer to the punch line.

During that sleepless night, which had become early morning, Dencil worked alone at the draftsman's table, sketching and resketching the Pixler mansion renderings, making redemptive changes possible even though construction was well underway. Looking over his shoulder as though someone were watching, Hobby stooped to consult the works of others for revisions to the disaster. The rows of architectural texts and design books displayed around him were meant to be exactly that: only displays, not actually reference books, especially for a professional architect of his celebrity. However, at that point Hobby Dencil was mentally drained and truly frustrated, his self-persecution over the whole Cordell and Rachel ordeal preventing any of his creative architectural juices from flowing naturally. He needed some help with brainstorming.

"Maybe she'll consent to this." Dencil fought a mental referral to Mrs. Pixler in the manner of the joke heard earlier on the radio. "I'll add this Flemish bond brickwork here and throw in some fanlights," he said as he marked the drawings. "If we could just include a few Federal influences to tone down the rest of this mess," he begged aloud in prayer as he finished a fourth cup of black coffee, the beverage no longer hot but still caffeinated. Hobby eliminated the term *Fantasy Room* from the drawings of what would be a den for most normal people and renamed the room *Garden* as it was meant, although a change in nomenclature would not abolish Rachel's ostentatious decorative choices.

Next, Dencil reworked the location and configuration of the library without revising any plumbing or major electrical designs. He then corrected that label as well while obliterating the thick interior wall masonry the madam had demanded, which looked like nothing more than expensive stucco. Even she had recognized the futility of shaping the material into his and her statuettes, not meant as anatomical replicas of the lord and lady of the manor, but intended to be more abstract. Rachel Pixler had taken some sculpting classes at the art museum and had planned to lend her own artistic legacy to the house, choosing the library (or as she preferred to call it, the 'Meditation Gallery') for the monuments. Fortunately for Dencil and anyone else who was destined to enter the room, Mrs. Pixler failed the class and dropped the idea.

Frantically reworking the design and taking advantage of the room's three exposures, he cleared the area where the busts of the couple were to rest on pedestals, forever guarding the opulence of the Pixler success. "More like standing in effigy!" he blurted as he turned another page. Believing the statues forever banned from the library, the frantic architect found valuable space for a window and much needed natural lighting. "I'll work that window into the façade somehow," he decided.

It was nearly 5:30 a.m. Dencil had been at work for more than three hours, trying to push the architectural revisions to the limit. "How much gaudiness could anyone want!" he shouted at his university diploma, framed expensively in triple mat and brought from his main office in Memphis to hang proudly on the wall before him, void of even a speck of dust. "I should have quit this damn job long ago," he shouted even louder at the certificate as though to shield it from the shame he had brought his mentors. As he continued to make alterations that he hoped would slide by the Pixlers, Dencil proceeded to add a domed ceiling to another room while removing the terra cotta wall panels embedded with intricate foliage designs. He then scaled down the passageway between the living room and the hall and revised the millwork, calling for classical moldings with wooden baseboards. Stenciling the wooden floors to parallel the ceiling design would be a stretch, but the caffeine of a fifth cup was starting to get to him.

Even in the rear hall, Rachel had demanded stairs with an ornate balustrade which Dencil doubted would ever be graced by anyone but the maids, maintenance staff, or other employees not using the back elevator. "No one who counts will ever see this space," Hobby decided aloud as he skipped any revisions to the rear stairwell. "Leaving that hellashush nightmare alone will be a bargaining chip for fixing the rest of this."

Hobby stopped drawing and printing for a minute, letting his pencil roll from his cramped fingers. *This is not what I wanted, Hobby! It's not what my husband – what we – are paying you for, Hobby!* he imagined as Rachel's reaction to the changes in progress. In contrast, sometimes the immature woman's mind seemed preoccupied during their discussions, and Hobby again prayed that this next encounter would not be a true butting of heads. Except for the psychedelic floor, Dencil had resolved all his concerns with the Meditation Gallery.

"Maybe I can cover that hellish floor with a cut-down from the European carpet I used a few months ago. I know that wonderful piece will be ample," he rambled on. "It will make a great Dhurrie and add some much-needed antique flair to the library," he reassured himself with relief. Early on in the working relationship with Mr. and Mrs. Cordell Pixler, Dencil had sensed a deep-seated insecurity in Rachel's quest for one-upmanship. The architect's dissection of the psyche of Rachel Pixler had been precise, and he knew immediately that he had devised an appealing solution to mask the hideous floor. Once she learned that a certain house in Dallas shared the same expensive floor covering, she would be thrilled, but never admit the sentiment.

Anyway, it would soon all be over, the reason for his insomnia. In fewer than six weeks, even with the modifications before him included, the architectural design aspect of the Pixler Palace project would be complete. At last he would be free, leaving the building contractor to fend for himself in finishing the construction. Hobby shuddered at the thought of the detailed punch list Rachel Pixler would compile for the tortured contractor. That would be a horrific nightmare all its own.

By strict intent, the contract between the Pixlers and Hobby Dencil and Associates absolved the architect of any responsibility for the quality of the building's construction, as well as for any engineering faults exposed during the six months after completion date. The manner in which the bricks were laid, the mortar poured, or the nails driven were issues directly tied to construction, not design. "That sucker contractor and that joker of a landscape architect will be left to pick up the pieces ... the Pixler pieces," he laughed deliriously, more from relief than the exhaustion of the hour. "Once that damned atrocity is turned over to those two guys, this job for me will be over forever, except for consultation over a few interior touch-ups." As Dencil leaned back as far as the stool to his draftsman's table would allow, he cheered his diploma, "In a few weeks I'll be free. Definitely Free! Yes!"

He and the cat would finally be able to sleep.

"Oh, my God!" Dencil screamed as he changed from jubilation to horror, rocking forward to reality on his stool with such thrust that pens and his sixth cup of coffee shook to the floor. "*Hobby Dencil* will forever be emblazoned on each brick, statue, four-by-four, painted molding and section of tacky tile."

He shook his head in bewildered grief and shame as he stared at his diploma. "I can't let this happen. I just can't."

Chapter
17

◆◆◆

THE DESSERTS

Understanding human nature had been expensive for The Foundation for the Furtherance of the Larkspur Institute for Education. That learned characteristic was attributed to hours of consulting work paid to an Atlanta firm kept on retainer. The trusting parents and students governed by that board would have expected no less from such an esteemed local group of veteran educators and successful business persons: omniscient, philosophical individuals who strove to maintain the status quo for their student progeny while making token efforts at progress. Citing other commitments, Cordell Pixler declined his freshman appointment to that educational board but recommended that his wife be anointed in his place. Consequently, Rachel Pixler promptly landed a spot on the illustrious panel, her husband's financial reputation in the community having made her a shoo-in choice for the selection committee.

Eugene "Nookie" McNabb was the president of The Foundation for the Furtherance of the Larkspur Institute for Education. The origin of the nickname *Nookie* was never fully explained, but the title graduated with him from Ole Miss and was later dropped in respectable circles. McNabb's naming a Pixler to the educational board was not meant merely to bestow an honor on a wealthy attorney or a would-be socialite. There was other motive.

Likewise, the incentive for Rachel Pixler's selection was neither a consolation prize meant to placate her husband nor the reason associated with the derivation of McNabb's nickname. Perpetuation of the foundation's agenda and its continued prominence in social circles was of extreme importance, at least in the eyes and mind of its president. And a Pixler as the newest board member was part of that principal goal.

The foundation's annual fundraiser had become a highlight of the spring party circuit in Larkspur. A demanding crowd expected each installment to top the previous one. Location choices had dwindled during the years, the elaborate houses or plush restaurants becoming either too small or too often frequented to be considered a real draw for the high price of admission – simply not special enough. Being the principal investor in the Rexford Hotel, the board president would have proposed staging the event in his own illustrious establishment except that the restaurant and its moderately-sized attached convention hall had been utilized in the preceding year.

No one on the foundation's board, particularly not its president, would tolerate a stale or ho-hum attempt at a soiree. Eugene McNabb hoped, in fact, literally prayed daily, that the upcoming attempt at raising money would be at least as successful as in the past. While the institute was in no way destitute, as it never had been, simply keeping the coffers overflowing would guarantee his reelection as president of the board.

For Eugene "Nookie" McNabb there was indeed an answer to those repetitive prayers in the person of Mrs. Cordell Pixler.

During a coffee and dessert break from one of her initial meetings as a freshman board member, the president motioned

Rachel aside. From a corner near the buffet table, he commented, "I'm sure your new home will be charming indeed, Rachel," he said, smiling enthusiastically. "It certainly looks exquisite from the exterior." That comment was more than a polite stretch. The house was not exactly to McNabb's taste but nonetheless would satisfy a throng of the town's curiosity seekers. "When I drove by it the other day it seemed almost completed," he continued while stirring in an artificial sweetener, the brand in the yellow packet. "I know you and Cordell are excited, just dying to move in."

"Oh, ah, well, of course." Rachel still felt a bit uncomfortable about her seat on the board. She was younger than the other members, although there were a few other females. Compounding her awkwardness was the knowledge that she was first runner-up in McNabb's selection process. "The landscaping is going in later this week, Mr. McNabb, as soon as the outdoor lighting is completed. They're having to install larger electric breakers because the first box went up in a puff of smoke when they did a dry run lighting the nightscape. The chief electrician didn't want to mess up the grass and plants with a lot of extra digging to bury more wires."

"The electrician probably asked the landscape foreman to hold up with the plantings for a bit. There's always something when you're building, some doggone delay, especially with a place as wonderful as yours," McNabb smiled. "And I know you and your husband want it to be just perfect."

Rachel nodded politely, again with an anxious air as she bit into a vanilla petit four, holding a paper napkin under her chin to catch the crumbs. She had chosen vanilla over the chocolate.

"And, of course, everyone will want to see your home, even without landscaping." McNabb hesitated slightly although he fully anticipated that Rachel Pixler would jump at the ensuing suggestion. "You know, we've been waiting for just the right spot to hold our school's annual fundraiser."

"Well, ah, I ... "

"Hosting such a worthwhile affair would be such an outstanding tribute to the community. Your house will be a showplace, a real showplace! And, like I just said, everyone in Larkspur and the surrounding area will want to see it. I expect the draw could include all of North and Central Mississippi, maybe even up to Memphis and West Memphis. The foundation has patrons all over the place, and I'll bet they're dying to see your breathtaking home." McNabb sometimes surprised himself with his feigned sincerity.

Of course, Rachel was thrilled at the suggestion but somehow forced a modest response as she swallowed the last bite of her dessert and mocked a blushed surprise. "Gosh, that's so sweet of you to offer to let me, let us, open our home for the school. What an honor for me, for Cordell and me, I mean!"

Smugly, the president faked surprise at her taking the bait. His initial smile of gratification then fell like a lead balloon as the young Mrs. Pixler shocked him back to a humility he seldom experienced.

"But I guess I should discuss this with my husband first. I'm not sure that he ... "

"Tickets to an event at your fabulous house will sell like hot cakes, like hot cakes!" Eugene "Nookie" McNabb interrupted in rising desperation, startling Rachel. "We might even be able to raise the admission price this year if we hold it at the Pixler ... (he almost said 'Pixler Palace') ... at your magnificent, new house." McNabb was certain that both elements, lots of countable money from volumes of ticket sales and a rousing good time for all, would be satisfied with an evening celebration at the Pixler property. The mansion was truly a residential structure never seen before in the Larkspur area, a structure that would attract the envious as well as those disdainful of overt pomp and circumstance, truly tacky ostentation.

The board president was no longer actually looking at Rachel
Pixler. He was looking through her, no, past her. He could
imagine the future smile on the school board treasurer's face, an
accountant by trade, sitting in a quiet room with a large number-
keyed calculator. A true bean counter, the treasurer would
gleefully reconcile the books following a flourishing fundraiser
at the Pixler Palace. That mountain-high pile of money would, of
course, satisfy the president's supporters and assure McNabb a
perpetual governing seat. A night of entertainment never before
seen in Larkspur would cement his re-election bid; McNabb was
convinced of it.

Thank God for the excesses of Cordell Pixler and his wife.

Surprising even herself with the voiced reluctance to accept
McNabb's idea, Rachel suddenly exuded an air of practicality over
the prospect of donating the use of her home. "You know, Mr.
McNabb, I'm really not sure what Cordell will think about all this.
When I discuss this proposal with him, he'll want to know more
than a few details."

While making the pitch to Mrs. Cordell Pixler, McNabb had
brimmed a china cup with hot coffee drawn from a silver urn on
the food service table. The first sip felt abruptly ice cold as his
lips mimicked the same tremor of aggravation shown in his hand.
"What kind of details?" he managed to respond with forced, steady
speech while keeping the coffee cup just as balanced.

"Like, how many people will be coming; will there be any
expenses on our behalf, expected or unexpected; who assumes the
liability of having all those people in our home – you know, who's
responsible if something happens or somebody gets hurt. After all,
you are aware that Cordell's a lawyer."

The formality of her questions was shocking to the president,
whose stomach by then had assumed the tremble from his hand
and cup. He had misjudged Rachel Pixler as a superficial airhead;
nevertheless, he continued to treat her that way.

"No need to worry about expenses, my dear," he retorted, struggling to maintain the upper hand in the high-stakes persuasive argument. In his opinion the Cordell Pixlers had more money than God and should skip concern over trivialities. "Well, ah, you see, all the food and drink will be donated, of course. The restaurants and liquor stores will be crawling over themselves, trying to outdo each other with their products. They'll be dying to participate in this fundraiser just to get wrapped up in all the publicity. I wouldn't be surprised if *Architectural Digest, Southern Living, Veranda, or Southern Accents* doesn't show up for a photo shoot. Heck, all four might just materialize." McNabb began to worry that he was stretching the hype to the point that even the likes of Rachel Pixler might believe impossible. "And no doubt their magazine editors will want personal interviews with you and Mr. Pixler."

Rachel listened intently; the word *publicity* was an attractive word, an exciting word. Also *photo shoot* had a nice ring.

"And since your home is going to be so accommodating, there'll be plenty of space for a really large group, certainly a gorgeous group, expecting a great time and all for a truly worthwhile cause – the education of the finest minds in our area." He forced a tear, then blotted it with the shirt sleeve covering his free left arm.

The strained melodrama of the president's presentation and its accompanying histrionics were lost on Mrs. Pixler and were actually unnecessary. The mention of the magazine coverage and the description of the attractive attendees hailing from beyond the bounds of Larkspur were irresistible. Rachel knew she had to have this party. She could envision the multi-page color spread in *Architectural Digest*, smiling to herself and even thinking about Hobby Dencil's presumed delight over such. Cordell would be flattered as well since few southern attorneys were similarly recognized. Anyway, it was her house even though Cordell was paying for it. She had worked for it and had put up with a lot, and he owed her for that. Cordell's opinion or approval of this gala was not really important, not really necessary. Her husband had his career. She was going to have this house and use it as she deemed fit. She was going to have this party.

Rachel's look was distant, quiet, as her mind raced. She had picked up another petit four, this time a chocolate one, and bit deeply into the confection, apparently in similar thought. McNabb's uncertainty over landing the Pixler deal was growing with each moment of her silence, with each bite of that dessert. He had made his best impromptu effort by going to the core of any would-be socialite's vanity. Waffling over such a commitment to donate the use of her new home was an abominable atrocity in his opinion. Eugene wanted to grab the rest of Rachel's petit four and cram it down her throat or better yet, shake Mrs. Pixler by the neck until her face turned the color of the chocolate. McNabb glanced around the room nervously as she chewed in front of him, seeing no other board member who might be able to talk some sense into the ingrate.

The board president began to suppose that maybe his group had been mistaken in appointing Rachel to the position of community member-at-large. Regarding the importance of superior education for Larkspur's youth, she was just too dense to see the big picture. He thought that possibly he should drop the idea and explore other options, particularly since her house was not yet completed. Besides, even though the construction was in its final stages, something could go wrong and the move-in date delayed.

Eugene McNabb chose not to give up and with renewed vigor continued to pitch the proposal. "Mrs. Pixler, please, this will be the most festive affair we have ever put together. There'll be dancing ... everyone will want to dance outside on your back patio surrounding the pool. We have always hired a live band, a much sought-after one, and this time will be no exception." There was no need for Rachel Pixler to have mentioned having a pool or a patio because McNabb had walked the property unhindered with his dog on several occasions, carefully inspecting the construction's progress.

Rachel seemed to be listening and absorbing as she swallowed the last morsel of chocolate petit four. Encouraged, McNabb continued. "All of the lucky attendees will get their money's worth under the stars, surrounded by outstanding dance music. Nothing will seem stale or stuffy like some other past events held in museums and ... "

"We'll be happy to do it! I know Cordell will be thrilled," she interrupted the monotonous persuasion, mercifully silencing McNabb's efforts which had approached begging.

The president's relief was released in a belabored exhale. Despite the fact that his coffee had grown truly cold, he swallowed a large gulp but wished for something much stronger.

Knowing she could handle her husband, Rachel had not needed any of McNabb's continued persuasion. She also was not stupid, not really, and she knew how to manage Cordell. Here was an opportunity that could reach beyond a few color magazine pictures or a local television interview. Observing the nearly frantic manner of the older gentleman before her, she realized that she could handle him as well. Rachel began, "We – the board that is – might have a real opportunity here. I believe my husband's interest in promoting the school will be awakened by this little project."

"I don't quite follow, Mrs. Pixler. Or, may I call you *Rachel*?"

"Sure, Eugene," she answered without missing a beat. "At our last board meeting we were discussing the addition of a new music and arts center for the school, even tossing around possible names for the building complex." With a linen napkin Rachel began to dab the chocolate icing remnants from her steady lips.

"That's correct. We spent nearly the entire meeting on that topic. However, there's this matter of the fundraiser. The board's got to make a decision about the annual ... "

"I know. I understand your concern. Ummm, let's see. What might sound nice? How can we guarantee a firm foundation for that much needed cultural center, a financial foundation, that is? What would accomplish that?"

"I don't follow quite follow you."

"Well, follow this. What might guarantee that the Larkspur Institute for Education gets that cultural center? Maybe a name for the place like ... Wait! I think I have it. Let's see ... the *Cordell and Rachel Pixler Center for the Advancement of Music and Culture.* Has a nice ring to it, don't you think, Eugene? Or maybe you would prefer the names reversed, Mr. President," she added with a sly, smiling titter that parted her full, pouty lips, the softness of which was a startling, unnerving contrast to her perfectly white, nearly sharp teeth. McNabb was uncertain which made him more uncomfortable.

His cell phone rang. That generic, irritating ring, the same ring one hears everywhere – in the checkout line of a store, sometimes intrusively in a theater, or constantly while walking through the mall – at anytime, in any crowd, even in a men's room, that incessant ring, moving up and down the range of musical tones, crescendo and decrescendo, touching nearly every decibel before the caller's intended mercifully answers and terminates the sound.

Wayne Simmons jerked the cell phone from his pocket and hit *SILENT*. He loathed being the center of any attention and softly cursed himself for not keeping the ring settings to *VIBRATE*. Nevertheless, no one around seemed to notice as he answered the call and ducked into a shady corner of the park, out of the way of the joggers and brisk walkers. He was in Memphis for a job, a successful one near the zoo. He usually left town quickly after an engagement, paying cash for a bus ticket or using the train if available. He knew there were security cameras in those places, some visible and some invisible. But a taxi or rental car was too great a risk, much easier to trace, he thought.

Although he never watched much television, he knew from crime dramas that telephone calls, even wireless ones, were easily traced and that detailed records of calls were kept by the communication companies. Wayne thought about keeping one of those disposable, temporary, cell phones with a pay-as-you-go plan. However, his clientele was built upon a growing list of gratified customers who passed his cell phone number along to others needing his services. So to keep that stream flowing, he had to keep the same cellular number to remain accessible. The highest level of self-confidence kept Wayne Simmons in business, a sense of self-admiration and a motto of *no job too big or too small*. Rarely had he refused a commission although he asked few questions, his one condition being that the situation not involve loss of life, at least not intentionally.

A fascination with fire and his ability to control it undetected was a driving force for Wayne Simmons. To that end, Simmons visited convenience stores after a job to check newspaper coverage for any suspicion of arson; seldom did he find mention of such. His self-esteem was boosted further by the omission of arson on local radio or television news programs. Whatever the news source, he delighted in the obligatory statements from the local fire inspectors or fire marshal – never any notion of foul play or at least none admitted. Even if they suspected a crime, Wayne knew that with a Simmons fire the authorities would by no means be able to prove it, much less solve it. Wayne Simmons was good, really good.

"Yeah, I'm here," he answered, flipping open the phone once more and silencing the annoying ring. He glanced around and without surprise noted no one looking in his direction. This self-perception of complete anonymity, as though he were a completely faceless nobody, was deep-seated and continued to serve him well professionally by squelching the paranoia of discovery. Such fear could cost him commissions.

Simmons' outward physical likeness matched his own self-image of banality: slight physique, average height, bland complexion, and colorless thin hair that blended easily into a crowd of people or actually into a group of anything. This sense of being ordinary in appearance in no way affected his professional opinion of himself but had indeed transposed into a nonchalant attitude toward detection regarding the traceability of cell phone records.

Once after a job in Alabama, Wayne watched a television detective show, one that had the word *law* in it and seemed to play two or three times a week in some form. A particular episode centered on solving a case using computer records of telephone calls. "Hell, I'd just burn the friggin' thing up. That'd take care of them friggin' records," he ruled while unscrewing the top to a longneck and hurling the cap to bounce off the television screen.

This cavalier attitude regarding communications extended to his customers. The phone calls were kept short and sweet, and he never questioned the source of any client referral. His was a specialized profession, advertising by word-of-mouth only with his cell number remaining within a tight circle. After all, his satisfied clients themselves wanted to remain shrouded in a cloak of confidentiality guaranteed by no written records. As long as the agreed upon payment for his professional services was waiting for him in cash as instructed, the client details were history.

Occasionally his pyrogenic expertise and ingenuity amazed even him. Examples were the crumbling, rat-infested building in Biloxi and the outdated condo in Gulfport, Mississippi. Since both fires were concurrent with Hurricane Katrina, the arson was camouflaged by the coincidental effects of the storm. Nonetheless, Wayne took all the credit, leaving none to nature but was thankful of his pre-pay policy.

Ever since he had finished high school, business had been good for Wayne Simmons, but he was sure he deserved it.

The call there in the park initially annoyed him since the caller ID feature on his cell phone read only *PRIVATE*. He usually ignored such calls: but as the phone continued its annoying chime, he was distracted by a young piece poured into hip-hugger jeans, bending slightly at the waist to get a drink from a nearby water fountain. Almost reflexively, Wayne flipped open his phone as the teenager ran her palms up and down her buttocks – long, slender, massaging fingers brandishing gaudy stone rings. Wayne imagined other of her body parts that might sport jewelry, tender areas pierced with petite gold bands that he wanted to touch and fondle.

Finding the client's voice deliberate with a tone of urgency, Simmons was startled into realizing that he had taken the unidentified call. The job sounded extremely important as the caller's request was for total destruction of the property and at a particular time. Wayne quoted a higher than usual fee because he perceived the potential client's expectations. After all, he had begun to realize that the people who contacted him were not shopping around for the best deal. His services were usually a last resort to solving a problem, and the needy clients would pay well.

The solicitation ended as usual with Wayne Simmons in control – payment details (amount of advance payment-in-full as well as method and place of drop-off) all determined and dictated by Wayne. From the caller's description, it was a large project located in a populated residential area – a new house, a big one, but he knew that the work could still be simple, in fact easy for

Wayne Simmons. The difference in this gig was its location – his hometown.

Since his mother died, the arsonist had not been back to the Larkspur area except for the easy job with the backyard propane tank. However, given this new opportunity he decided to devote more time to the advance site visit. Nothing really remained there for him, no parents and no siblings. In fact, he was sure that no one in the miserable town would remember him, much less recognize him.

The site inspection involved a ride around the target's neighborhood made with a level of curiosity, even with a hint of déjà vu. Of the few buddies he had at the private high school, most had been locked into the same orbit: a revolution of futile education, a perception of an unhappy home life dominated by a bastardly parent or parents, some low-paying job after graduation, and escapism through guzzling alcohol at any opportunity. He and his long-forgotten classmates had cruised Manorwood Heights, decorating the expansive, manicured lawns with uncrushed beer cans because crushing them would have required effort. An occasional quart-sized beer bottle tossed like a newspaper or a frisbee would hit a driveway selected at random, although the following morning the owners would assume differently.

Now several years later, the neighborhood appeared much the same, although daylight brought new perspectives. During those reckless adolescent meanderings through Manorwood Heights, Wayne thought little of the surroundings. The area was appreciated only as a quiet roadway interlacing expansive, solemn houses no doubt filled with snobby, rich folks waited on hand-and-foot by equally snobby servants. However, on this return to Manorwood he inconspicuously drove through the area at just below the speed limit in an effort to read the street names courtesy of the slower speed and daylight. Names ending in *Cove,*

Way, Court, Peak, or *Crest* blended with others such as *Run, Bend, Pointe*, or *Walk* as though someone had chosen the latter nomenclature group in remembrance of a country club exercise class. *Hunter's Pass* brought a smile to Simmons because the few houses on the short dead end were pink and yellow.

Just as in high school, Wayne Simmons still perceived the significant houses and streets in the neighborhood as frigid and uninviting, far different than the section of town where he lived with his late mother. Attending the private academy in Larkspur with the teenage elite who lived on these absurdly-named streets would have been out of reach for him financially had it not been for a scholarship. Mrs. Simmons had written the qualifying essay on her son's behalf although he was forced to go before a panel of Veterans' League judges – a lot of questions about patriotism, hard work, and belief in God. The contest had been a new one meant to honor deserving children of Vietnam War veterans, and somehow Wayne bluffed his way through. The grant would remain in effect through graduation provided that a B average remained in force as well. But to win the scholarship the veteran's story had to be filled with woe and financial depravity. The Simmons family met all qualifications.

Wayne Simmons' father indeed had been one of those woeful, unfortunate veterans. Although he had been decorated for outstanding service to his country during the Vietnam War, he returned to Mississippi with issues, mental issues. Appearing emotionally balanced at first, Wayne's dad nevertheless arrived from combat essentially unemployable, unable to maintain a job for more than a few months at a time due to flashbacks of horrific jungle scenes in Southeast Asia, or something like that.

More than ten years later would bring the birth of Wayne, somewhat of an unexpected gift to his parents who had believed that they would never have children. Mr. Simmons soon died of alcohol and cigarettes, as well as other extracurricular activities, while his widow continued to work in a local manufacturing plant. Wayne managed to stay in school and scrape up a *B* average though the Veterans' League looked the other way when he barely passed during his senior year.

The Vietnam Vet scholarship to Larkspur Christian Academy had been his mother's dream, not Wayne's. Mrs. Simmons had hoped to improve her child's life, catapult him into some sort of superior situation that the local public school could not offer. But her efforts were wasted, maybe even had backfired. Attending classes at what would become the Larkspur Institute for Education had been his only connection to a school that, from the outset, he found cold, even cruel at times. (A member of the drill team stopped him in the hall on his third day there and whispered in his right ear, "Why don't you slither on back to Larkspur High?") That sort of welcome as well as more subtle unkind student remarks or glances had made it impossible for Wayne to develop a sense of oneness with the private school. On the other hand, Mrs. Simmons' son had no problem with his life now; he remained completely satisfied in his adult career, continuing to lurk in the shadows as he did in high school.

Chapter
18
•••
THE ASSISTANT

"This one could have been a head scratcher."

Business had been fairly brisk for the Larkspur Fire Department, and with all the practice, I was getting pretty good at being a firefighter. As I looked and behaved less and less like a rookie, Fire Marshal Lisenbe seemed to be giving me greater responsibilities with each call, sparing many of the nuisance ones. It is surprising how many times a relatively small-town fire department is called to retrieve keys locked within cars of soccer moms and dads.

Over the next several months Alvin Coakley remained on staff as a fire investigator, inviting me to follow him around to the aftermath of most of the bonfires, the heavy stuff, and I accepted. As far as I could tell from my shadowing, he was excellent at inspecting fire scenes. His manner of investigation seemed almost clairvoyant at times. Yet, particularly in the beginning, I considered myself such a novice that it would not have taken much to impress me.

"Wonder why there's a pile of torched debris in the middle of this kitchen, a kitchen that's 'sposed to be empty since nobody lived here when the place burned?" Coakley continued as we both walked around the remnants of the room. The area had been on the east side of what was once a habitable house that had stood vacant for as long as anyone could remember, its fate now sealed by yesterday's inferno when I had the day off. Located in a section of Larkspur in which a real estate boom never happened, the long-suffering structure had even been overlooked by Habitat for Humanity and other community restoration efforts. Proudly occupying the front yards of surrounding homes were tireless cars elevated on blocks hidden from view by tall, wild grasses, all of which did nothing to help the area's desirability.

The charred sink resting in a corner atop cinders of cheap composite wood cabinets made it clear that the room Coakley was inspecting had once served as the kitchen. A few twisted pipes peeking from some blackened floorboards were additional obvious clues. "To make a long story short, I guess there could have been some stuff left in here when this place went up, you know, if the last tenants had been sort of sloppy and moved out in a hurry. Maybe they still owed for the rent," he answered himself since he knew that I was not going to respond. I had no clue as to why the debris would have been there in the center of the room or, for that matter, what difference the finding made in the scheme of things.

"Did the fire start here in the kitchen?" I asked, almost afraid to interrupt his train of thought.

"Well, I don't want to sound rude but there's no way. A fire wouldn't originate in the middle of a room, not on its own. And especially if there are no appliances around. And I don't see anything here that looks like what's left of an appliance." Coakley was trying to teach me a lesson in Fire Investigation 101: a fire originating in the center of a kitchen floor would have been extremely rare. Even I could see that the floor in the center of the room showed signs of intense heat that seemed to dissipate as the flames spread peripherally.

Suddenly I felt ignorant around Coakley, although that was not his intention. Even I could surmise that the ashes and charred material lying in the middle of the room had not been appliances or other types of electrical equipment. That type of low-end house would not have had features such as a serving or cooking island positioned near the center of its kitchen.

The holes in the burned ceiling and roof caused by leaping flames emitted ample light for our investigative tour, a narrative of which was documented by Coakley on a handheld digital recorder. With great precision he pointed his slim, black, high-powered flashlight toward the darker corners, searching throughout the structure for evidence of natural or unnatural causes of combustion. At his command I worked as a dutiful assistant, using the department's multi-pixel digital camera to document anything assumed significant: the shape and orientation of smoke stains on any of the remaining sections of plastered walls, water marks left by my buddies at the department, exposed electrical wires, or broken window panes. As was his custom, Coakley chose not to utilize video in collecting evidence inasmuch as he was required to submit still photos with paper file reports.

As we progressed to the central hall of the forties-style home, Coakley and I found the corridor to the bedroom area impassable. Distorted rafters and other attic materials had tumbled down, making even cursory inspection of the subflooring impossible. Therefore, Coakley redirected the survey toward the living room. Continuing to take digital photographs at the command of his pointed right forefinger, I preserved each important observation as he recorded the narrative. We stopped at the rear of the living room, finding the closet there minus its back wall as a result of collapse during the fire. This artificial passage exposed the master bedroom.

"Ummmmm." Alvin stopped for a moment, peering across the

room as he directed the flashlight beam toward what remained of the far wall. "Whaddaya think that stuff is?"

The light traced a string of charred clothes, mostly thick ashes that resembled burned-out charcoal. "Looks like what was once a pile of tee shirts," I answered as he moved closer, treading carefully across the room with the assistant following on the heels of the teacher and hoping that Coakley had correctly judged the strength of the remaining floor.

"Wonder what ignited those clothes?" Certainly his inquiry was directed toward thin air although I chose to attempt an answer.

"From the looks of what's left of that electrical outlet over there, it's possible that some short or spark or something like that ignited the pile of clothes." Alvin's facial expression failed to change during my theorizing, his genteel manner preventing an immediate counterpoint. So I continued, "Well, uh, mainly if the stuff had been lying around for awhile undisturbed, you know, really old clothes that could have been really dry, really combustible, so even a small spark from that outlet could have caused ... "

"Pardon me, I don't want to seem rude, but the electricity to this house wasn't hot when it burned. Hasn't been turned on for months, several months."

I decided not to respond, instead just snapped lots of pictures of the room.

"Let's see. This way into the bathroom," Coakley motioned with his flashlight as we walked carefully around the torched four-by-fours and entered the small bathroom. It had been lined with small black and white tiles, a decorative touch which seemed incongruous with the rest of the house, or what was left of it. Against the wall opposite the door was the bathtub, one of those four-legged cast iron antiques. Alvin lowered his face toward the rim of the blackened tub and sniffed.

"What are you doing?"

"Sniffing."

"That's what I thought."

Coakley ran his forefinger around the base of the tub's interior and put it to his lips and nostrils. "Yep, that's it."

"That's what?"

"Gas. Gasoline."

His determination was reached because no sign of flames leapt from the barrel of the tub to reach the ceiling, the bathtub having been marred by smoke and ash but not fire. Coakley put all the pieces together. "I know what you're thinkin'. To make a long story short – what they did, you see, was soak those clothes out there in this tub filled with gasoline." He jerked the flashlight back toward the bedroom at the pile of what I had surmised were remnants of old cotton tees. "And then they moved the clothes drenched in gasoline out into the bedroom, placing them at the wall near the electrical wall outlet. Did a fairly good job, though, and left no dribbling gasoline trail.

"The jokers thought that we wouldn't be surprised to find old clothes left lying around in a dump like this," he continued to assume correctly. "That's why they stashed that stuff so close to the electrical outlet. They figured that if there was an investigation then we would be stupid enough to think that the nearly seventy-year-old wiring simply shorted out, you know, maybe from an electrical surge that sparked that pile. The problem with that plan is like we said – *no electrical supply to the house.*"

Coakley cackled aloud at the idiocy of the perpetrator or perpetrators. As did I, the amateur effort had overlooked the electric meter still mounted on a remaining outside wall, the meter as dead now as it had been at the time of the fire. Seeming to ignore my erroneously-voiced suspicions about the fire's point of origin, Coakley somehow pitched his derogatory laugh only toward the unknown arsonists. I too laughed at the idiot or idiots, though with a hint of embarrassment.

We moved back to the kitchen, where he stood over the burned debris left in the center of the room. Coakley scooped up some of the thick ash with his right hand and sniffed the material as well. "Hard to tell sometime," Alvin said between short sniffs that would have initiated sneezing for most individuals.

"Hard to tell what?" I had decided it best simply to ask questions and offer no further opinions.

"Sometimes the combustion will be so intense that the fuel smell is disguised. To make a long story short, betcha those jokers first soaked this material in the bathtub, you know, planning a kitchen fire before deciding to disguise their little game as electrical." Coakley repeated this assumption into the recorder, rephrasing his wording professionally in the form of a determination. I took some more pictures and decided then that maybe I should go back to those MCAT prep books – maybe pick up the new editions and forget the fire stuff.

"As soon as those two pay their final bill I'm going to get a new cell phone number," he wryly told his secretary weeks later; to him it had seemed years. As she lowered her head slightly, glancing away from the computer screen past the top of her glasses, Telly King's facial muscles tightened around her lips. Sensing an uncharacteristic degree of excitement in her employer's demeanor, the secretary molded her mouth into more than its usual pursed shape. This expression exuded the annoyance of being interrupted, an annoyance that was certain to go ignored by her boss. Since her retirement from the math department at the institute, Telly had been employed part-time working for Hobby Dencil since he had temporarily relocated his office to Larkspur from Memphis.

The job at Dencil and Associates consisted of weekday mornings only and seldom required duties traditionally associated with a secretary inasmuch as Hobby Dencil sent few letters and received few landline calls. Much of her job consisted of entering client information into a simple computer program and posting payments for professional fees, mostly from the Pixlers. The former math teacher took her work seriously and strove to work efficiently, especially because she desired to devote no more hours to the architect than required by her original commitment. As Dencil spoke, Telly was completing the last financial entry for the morning and did little to disguise her annoyance over the interruption.

"Mr. Dencil, have you forgotten that appointment in Montclair? You agreed to meet with the doctor right after lunch today at 1:30. Let's see. That's right – 1:30," King asserted as she checked Dencil's calendar on her computer program.

"Telly, I've asked you to call me *Hobby*. You've worked with me long enough. You really should think about moving to Memphis when I'm finally finished with that Godforsaken Pixler ... "

"Yes, I've double checked, Mr. Dencil. Your appointment with that doctor is at 1:30, and since she's called several times to confirm it, I doubt if the lady expects you to be late. The doctor said something about wanting to add on a child's playroom, a really nice, large one."

"Child's playroom?" Hobby asked helplessly, not directing his disbelief at the office assistant but instead at the gods of architecture.

Telly highlighted the name *Dr. Aslyn Hawes* on the computer screen as the printer suddenly came to life, spitting out an appointment reminder for Dencil. "Here, Mr. Dencil. Here's the doctor's address and her phone number highlighted in bold, just in case you get lost once you get to Montclair."

While rising from her desk to leave, King grabbed her purse with her right hand and handed Hobby the printed sheet with her left. There was no eye contact as these maneuvers seemed to blend into one hurried motion, pushing her body to the exit. Telly was due at the agency by one o'clock, not to seek another job for herself but to report for her second part-time retirement occupation. Prior to the hurricane, working at the temp agency had been a real sleeper. However, the influx of evacuees from the Mississippi Gulf Coast and New Orleans had nearly overloaded the computer software files with job seekers. Consequently, Telly's duties as an employment counselor were no longer mechanical, no longer pure rote. Reviewing the applications before entering the information into a computer was well below interesting, rising only to an occasional level of fascination when the completed forms seemed replete with imaginary job history.

But she would find this next one seemingly sincere. The story was sad.

The woman had been waiting in the side chair of Telly's cubicle since 12:30 p.m.

"Hello, my I help you? I'm sorry that you've been waiting, but ... "

"That's okay. The receptionist told me that you didn't come in until one o'clock. You were the only counselor available, so I decided just to wait."

Telly set her purse in the lower right hand desk drawer. While she attempted to conceal the irritation of being pushed into work before a cup of coffee, the effort was transparent.

"Like I said, the woman at the front desk told me to wait here. Even though I was a little early for my appointment."

"Yes, ah, well, that's all right." To Telly the woman appeared attractive although beaten, not physically, but emotionally, exuding the appearance of defeat and utter disappointment. The applicant had completed the written form and nervously rolled the top right edge of the thick orange paper between her thumb and forefinger.

"Also, the woman at the front desk asked me to fill this out and give it to you. I really haven't worked much. I've been raising two girls."

After logging onto her desktop terminal, Telly reached over for the completed personnel application, skipping eye contact. As though on second thought, she glanced over to the client and smiled briefly with forced politeness. The woman was attractive, thick long red hair with a color much too intense to be unnatural. Her dress was just a notch above casual, typical for a former housewife attempting to enter the business world. Telly had seen it before.

She scanned the woman's information. No empty space was left unfilled. The information was neatly hand-printed with no crossed-out words or misspellings obvious at first glance. There was little paid work history to enter into the computer, mostly community service or volunteer activities. The *Marital Status* blank was marked *Widow* and that of next-of-kin was completed with the names of two females identified as daughters. Telly seldom inquired about the marital situation; there were so many divorces these days, resulting in the very reason this job placement company was guaranteed a steady stream of applicants. However, there were few forms with the *Widow* blank checked, particularly tagged to a fairly youthful applicant.

While Faith forced patience with the older woman as the computer keyboard entries seemed more involved than the handwritten paper version, her mind drifted away from the cubicle and the thinly upholstered office chair in which she sat. There was renewed regret over the primary reasons to be sitting across from the woman. Had the meager inheritance from her late husband survived the stock market, and their home Hurricane Katrina, and had her late sister's house in Larkspur been safely inhabitable or at least salable, then this appointment for Faith Behneman would never have been necessary.

Her mind raced in renewed circles of lament as she sat almost transfixed at the woman typing somewhat more rapidly now, accurately transferring each printed character of the completed form onto the computer screen. Faith noticed that this Mrs. Telly King would pause momentarily as though to stare at certain sections of her application, then reflect briefly on its contents before continuing to type away.

"I see that you have had experience in the catering business?" Halting the rhythm of her fingers as she looked over to Faith to speak, Mrs. King's inflection was not missed on Faith.

"You're correct. I ... " (Faith's self-destructive daydreaming was halted) " ... helped, I mean worked, on several fund-raising, I mean commercial, projects with my children's schools on the coast, where we used to live. One of the other mothers was a professional caterer and she taught me a lot, shared a lot of her secrets."

Faith noticed that Mrs. King sat expressionless.

"She was a really good caterer. Really good and really popular. Yes, she was. Hired for a lot of parties on the coast, even over in New Orleans, too, before the hurricane, that is. But her business is starting to pick back up now. Yes ... it really is." Faith Behneman had always been able to label a liar and wondered if this woman had the same gift.

"I see. Well, one of our strongest clients is in need of additional service staff for an important function in a few weeks. Our client is catering a gala at a new home here in Larkspur. It was just built by a lawyer and his wife."

"Right, I think I may have seen something about that in the newspaper yesterday." Faith's stomach turned one-hundred and eighty degrees as she thought about Attorney Cordell Pixler and what he had done to her sister. She forced a response. "The article said five hundred or more people were expected, I think."

"It's a fundraiser for the private school here in Larkspur." Telly was careful to provide that detail because she doubted an applicant for temporary employment would know much about an area private school. "You won't be doing any cooking, of course, but you'll be passing trays of food and picking up cups and glasses."

Faith sat motionless, the perfect stoic. In her opinion, the potential job placement was no more than that of a maid. But she needed something; she needed some money. She was tired of living in the extended stay motel all these months, and the FEMA housing funds had been long gone, as was the community pity. As she began to estimate the number of hours of employment this commission would assure, Mrs. King continued, "The pay is a couple of dollars more than minimum wage, but there'll be some sort of tip; I'm reasonably sure of it. Of course, our usual placement percentage will be withheld from your check, in addition to the standard tax deductions.

"I know it may not sound like much, but this is your first time with our agency. If things go nicely, if we get a good report from the client about your work, then I'm sure there'll be other placements. Maybe something every day, or better yet, long-term."

"What do you mean 'if we get a good report from the client about your work'?"

"I mean, if we don't get any complaints about you," Telly clarified.

"Oh, I can assure you, Mrs. King. You won't get any complaints about me."

It would have been impossible for any coherent person residing in or near Larkspur to be unaware of that upcoming event. Publicity about the fundraising gala at the lawyer's newly completed house had flooded the Larkspur media which touted it as a landmark event. Advance tickets were advertised at one-hundred fifty dollars per person or a bargain at two-hundred seventy dollars a couple. The unfortunates who chose last-minute attendance would pay two hundred per single or three hundred twenty-five per couple.

The Larkspur newspaper had unleashed a four-page color spread displaying the beautiful Pixlers, smiling with obvious and uncontrollable eagerness over sharing their gracious new home with the public. (Rachel had come to grips with most of Dencil's eleventh hour architectural changes, but held her ground on some.) Next to the nearly full-page photo of Cordell and Rachel Pixler were minor features about other Larkspur Institute volunteers, identified as sacrificing parents and painstaking fundraiser organizers. Adjacent to those smiles were placed the chefs, artists, authors, artisans, interior decorators, and gift shop owners who had jumped to donate their time and wares to the gallant money-gathering effort. Voluntary exclusion from that band of merchant-supporters would have earned permanent commercial blacklisting.

The local television stations would not be outdone by the print media. As Faith watched the news broadcasts, it was as though each anchor's ratings depended on the actual numbers attending the party. Photographs and video tours of the gala's planned backdrop were aired so frequently and in such detail that Faith assumed it possible to stroll through the Pixler mansion unescorted and find every toilet.

The lawyer's wife, a pretty blonde thing, had been interviewed by all three local television stations. Even one of the stations based in Memphis did a Sunday afternoon interview with the Pixlers, portraying the two as a fairytale couple devoted to opening their home in the name of education. Somehow CNN had skipped the opportunity.

During all the malpractice proceedings against that doctor who had killed her niece, Faith had never seen Mrs. Pixler, for there would have been no reason to meet her. While watching the laborious television features of the upcoming event, she decided that the woman beside the swindling lawyer was really just a girl, way too young for Pixler. Maybe she was a follow-up wife, or maybe she was herself a poster child for plastic surgery. But during the trial against that doctor – *what was his name anyway, Foxworth?* – Pixler had implied distaste for plastic surgery and plastic surgeons, but then Charity and she had learned much too late that he was a liar and a cheat.

As Faith sat in the temporary job placement office staring at the counselor, watching her lips move in instruction and hearing none of it, she thought about that doctor – the one justly degraded in court by the lawyer with the beautiful young wife, the doctor who murdered her niece and then indirectly killed her sister. She wondered if that doctor had owned a house as amazing as the lawyer's, but anyway it did not matter because the doctor and his own wife were dead.

"He probably did," she decided aloud about the dead doctor's house as Telly King looked up from the computer printer.

"I'm sorry, beg your pardon. Did you say something?" Mrs. King asked.

"No, ah, I didn't say anything." Faith grabbed her purse from the floor as it leaned against her chair. "Is this all I have to do?" she asked as she partially rose from the seat.

"Yes, here is the paperwork you'll need to give to the head caterer when you report Saturday." Telly handed the two freshly printed sheets to Faith Behneman, who suddenly seemed pale and at the same time angry. "Her name is Yvette. You won't be able to miss her. The location's address is at the top of the first page, but you'll ride in a van from the catering business. That address is at the bottom. Don't be late, please."

Faith took the papers and stood to leave, forcing a "Thank you."

Walking from the cubicle toward the front door, she stopped, turned, and stepped back toward the agent. "What time am I supposed to be there, and what do I wear?"

Puzzled, King replied curtly, "I just gave you your instructions, printed in black and white on those pages you are holding right there in your right hand with the time, date, location, and dress highlighted. Plus I went over them with you, one-by-one, just a couple of seconds ago."

"Well, I guess, I ... missed that."

"Well, I guess you did." Telly suddenly doubted the wisdom of placing this woman at such an important function, and then reasoned that maybe Faith Behneman was just overly distracted by financial worry. After all, she was reasonably attractive, had completed two years of college, and seemed to have good sense. At least she could complete an information form neatly and thoroughly. "If you can't come up with a caterer's uniform by Saturday, a clean, starched, white, and cotton one – you know, borrow one from a friend or something – Yvette will have a loaner for you. But only this once. You'll certainly need to have your own uniform if we use you again."

After studying Faith as though a store mannequin, Telly King added decisively, "Yes, I'm sure he'll have your size. You look to be about average."

Chapter
19

♦♦♦

THE ENCOUNTER

I did my best to visit him as often as possible even though the telephone summonses had dropped off, as though he had given up. The recurring image of my grandfather sitting alone in that walnut room, watching those old home movies while studying photos and scrapbooks, could drown a happy moment, even a stimulating one with Kaylee.

Shopping for steaks at the market was not one of those stimulating dates but soon developed into a downer, referencing my grandfather's existence. It was on the sushi isle where we ran into Linton Desselle.

"Well, hello, young man. How's our local hero, or has all that stuff worn off by now?"

Desselle really expected no answer. Granddad had once mentioned to me that this longtime golfing buddy's quest for superiority on the links had softened since his own grandchild had made medical school. Desselle had finally beaten Sheridan Foxworth, Sr., at something. The irony of Linton Desselle's self-determined winning of a round in life was that grandson Oby was smoldering toward the low end of the medical school grade curve, a fact that he may not have shared with his doting grandfather, a fact that really did not matter.

"Still playing much golf, Mr. Lin?" I asked as Kaylee inspected the fresh shrimp near me, planning to convert our meal to surf-and-turf. She seemed to have forgotten that a fireman's salary was paying the grocery bill.

She caught my stingy vibes and interrupted, "Don't worry, Baby. We'll go halvsies at check-out."

"Yes, I'm playing a fair amount, though I miss seeing your grandfather."

Without giving me an opportunity to question his comment about Granddad, he continued. "The Club has just added another nine over by the river. Did a really nice job of it. By the way, who is this lovely young lady with you?"

My breeding should have already led to an instant introduction of my girlfriend, but at that moment she had moved down the aisle behind us, gazing at the lobster tank as though she were at a pet shop. "Oh, yes, sir. Ah, this is Kaylee Lisenbe," I pointed as she walked back to us. Besides, his comment *miss seeing your grandfather* had thrown me.

"You're the fire marshal's daughter, I believe." As Linton Desselle extended his hand, Kaylee smiled and reciprocated while momentarily abandoning her study of crustaceans. "I'm sure your father is pleased to have this fine young man working for him," he added to her.

"Definitely," Kaylee responded as she withdrew her right hand from the completed handshake and reached for my waist. "I just wish this fine young man here did not have to spend so much time down at the fire station," she added with a light squeeze. "I guess the battle for his affections is going to get rougher when Sher starts on that med school prep course."

"Oh, I see." Desselle turned toward me almost in question. "I remember that you had tried to get accepted, I mean, had applied to the university medical school a few years ago. But I guess you changed your mind about going right then or something like that."

Who was he kidding anyway? Linton Desselle was fully cognizant of my dismal attempt at getting into medical school. He seemed to have forgotten that his own grandson's foray into med school had barely missed dismal, though you had to give him credit for eventually winning a coveted spot. Oby Desselle had made some wise choices at the correct times and had delayed his own pursuit of social contentment until first landing in med school. In college he seldom went out, but instead sucked up to the professors, participated in charitable community service, and served on student government committees: all the stuff the medical school committee treasures. Even with all that dedication, he was accepted first as an alternate, but at least he got in. But from what I had heard, once he was safely tucked away on the medical school roster, he rapidly made up for lost opportunities as he basked in the attention of a bragging grandfather.

Over the last several years my own grandfather had certainly not been blessed with any bragging rights. Standing there in the aisle of the meat market, that fact brought renewed sadness for me, actually guilt. Kaylee had encouraged me to give it another shot, but until now the discussions had been private. My girlfriend's sudden decision to announce my renewed interest in medical school was a surprising but nice counterpoint to Desselle's superior attitude.

Nevertheless, he seemed unscathed regarding my decision to reapply and retorted, "That's fine, Sher. But, let's see. What about your grades in undergraduate school? I remember Sheridan seemed to be really worried about your marks at Ole Miss, particularly during your freshman year. He mentioned it a few times over drinks in the Nineteenth Hole."

Despite practically being a stranger to Linton Desselle, Kaylee accurately accessed the undertones of the situation and rebounded on behalf of the Foxworth family. The degree to which she stood at allegiance was beyond that of a mere seasoned girlfriend; she was a true diplomat. "You know, Mr. Desselle, my guess is that the medical admissions committee likes maturity." Kaylee's opinions were indeed a guess although she remembered a few conversations with an opinionated cousin who had applied for medical school a few years previously. "A candidate who's been out in the work force for a few years might seem stable, more focused than some other students, and would stay that way."

Kaylee's comments were also a subtle revelation and criticism that would be missed on Mr. Desselle. On a recent night out, she and I had bumped into his grandson in a Jackson restaurant, an urban-oriented, eclectic place up the street from the medical center. Kaylee and I both had the next day off, a weekday, a luxury the medical school professors likely had withheld from Oby and his partying entourage. But that evening the younger Desselle seemed oblivious to concerns about microscopes, pharmacology, or professional physical exams as he repeatedly hit on and danced with various single girls in the bar. I had been to that establishment a couple of times before and had never found dancing to be one of the activities, probably because there was no featured music. That particular night between the permanent cocktail stations and the circulation of the waiters, Oby Desselle was making his own music as he occasionally even danced solo. When greeting my former high school classmate at the service bar during one of his refueling stops, his eyes initially appeared too glazed to recognize me. However, after placing his order he spoke with slurred familiarity.

"A top MCAT score will offset some of that GPA," Kaylee continued. "Sher is going to start that medical college admissions test review course in the next couple of months. They offer it up in Memphis. The schedule is flexible for guys like him who work, so he'll be able to handle it."

Desselle grinned partially in disbelief of my plans and also in embarrassment over the tight squeeze my imaginative, affectionate girlfriend had landed around my waist.

Actually Kaylee and I had only discussed the plans she detailed as final to Linton Desselle. A few days ago she downloaded the application for the med school prep course from the website and brought the print over to me. "Your dad may not appreciate your stealing away his best fireman and making it possible for the med school to snap me up," I responded then. "From the looks of things, I suspect he's grooming me as his successor," I joked that day, although from the ongoing attitude of Fire Marshal Lisenbe that had truly been my take on things.

Kaylee now had the floor, or maybe the aisle, during that impromptu meat market meeting with Mr. Desselle. She had taken an immediate dislike to the smug, older man whom she had just met, but he had no reason to reciprocate as of yet. I for one decided it best simply to remain silent and I did, stepping aside to allow Kaylee to approach Desselle cunningly, as though zooming in for the kill.

"And you know that college GPA is really not a dead issue. It's a label that everyone seems to be so worried about. In fact, Sher can still do something about it. He can take some of those bombed-out Ole Miss courses over and bump those grades right up!" Kaylee cried out with such excitement that two startled sushi customers looked our way with annoyance, then resumed their intense study of the treasured packages of izumadai, unagi, shiro maguro, and ankimo.

"They now have these intersession college courses," Kaylee continued unabashed, squeezing me tighter at the waist, "where

Sher can take something between semesters on sort of a fast track so that he won't have to miss much work. My dad would like that because Sher has done great in the fire department – has been a really fast learner, according to my dad."

Desselle was starting to appear rather uncomfortable. He had nothing in common professionally with Fire Marshal Lisenbe although he had shared a golf foursome with him on occasion.

"And, of course, there's always summer school." Kaylee added, preparing for her victorious climax to the argument that the grandson of Linton Desselle would not be the only young guy from Larkspur to attend med school. Her arguments for resurrecting my dismal efforts in that direction could not have been more positive had she been formally trained in debate. "Oh, yeah. There's another thing he's working on that will sound really top-notch during his medical school interview."

Desselle then redirected his gaze from the mission-driven, attractive young woman before him and instead stared at me as though to ask, "What is this? What now?"

I shrugged my shoulders with the same question, then tilted my head and jerked my eyes toward Kaylee, turning his attention back to Miss Lisenbe for the answers.

"A friend told me that the medical school admissions board, the people that interview those poor nervous applicants, are blown away when an interviewee has some medical experience – you know, has tested the waters."

I had never heard that any of the professors on the admissions board were ever 'blown away' by anything; they expected the applicants to be outstanding. A benchmark of excellence had been set for acceptance to medical school from which the judges merely subtracted the negatives, coming up with a class of would-be doctors as varied as the patients to be treated. I thought about Oby Desselle's 'testing the waters,' the firewaters at the bar in Jackson the other night. No telling what else he had tested.

Meanwhile, Kaylee seemed to be on a roll; where she was rolling, I was not sure.

"I talked with my own doctor the other day when I was over in Montclair," she continued. "Dr. Chamblee sponsors college and other students interested in medical careers – lets them do what's called *shadowing*. They get to follow him around for a few days, like when he goes to surgery and does hysterectomies, or whatever, and then watch when he delivers babies, that is, as long as the patients don't mind."

Kaylee was referring to her gynecologist, whom I had never met and really did not care to. She had mentioned him to me once in discussing her birth control, but other than that aspect of Dr. Chamblee I knew all I needed to know: his prescription had been reliable. I knew nothing of his mission to further the career choices of a few science-oriented students.

"Those kids just observe my doctor doing what he does to help people. Kind of lets the student get his or her feet wet, decide whether or not a medical career is the right fit."

I looked over at Mr. Desselle as he checked his watch.

"Next month Sher is going to spend some time over in Montclair with Dr. Chamblee before he starts his fellowship in reproductive endocrinology. Dr. Chamblee wants additional training in helping infertile couples have babies. I think he'll be good at that. " I felt a twinge of jealousy as Kaylee smiled proudly about her Dr. Knox Chamblee.

I fought successfully to mask my surprise over all of these revelations concerning my evolving career. Apparently Kaylee's driving mood that day in the grocery store was more than scoring one-upmanship over my grandfather's peer. In placing me in a situation that I could not deny, my girlfriend was renewing my quest toward medical school – not so far behind Oby's career that it could not be equaled or maybe even surpassed. There really was no rivalry between the young, prodigal Desselle and me and there certainly would never be, particularly if he continued his adult pursuit of transcendental nightlife.

My head had began to hurt, partially because I was hungry and had planned to already have the food on the grill by then, but mostly from the educational strategy to which Kaylee was publicly and almost unilaterally committing me. That obviously entailed an extensive, back-breaking prep course for the medical school admissions test and plans for me to follow a guy around while he destroyed my lasting adolescent appreciation for the female human body.

Desselle himself was shifting in position, clearly having heard more than he cared to and probably hungry as well. "Ahhhhh, it seems as though you two have an ambitious campaign ahead," he summarized, avoiding further eye contact as he planned an escape from Kaylee. Tossing his selection of steaks into the shopping cart as he turned it toward the exit, Linton Desselle added, "It's been nice meeting you Miss Lisenbe and visiting with you again, Sher. I better run these steaks home real quick before they spoil."

"Oh, yes, it was great meeting you also, Mr. Desselle," she responded, seemingly much more demure.

"Thank you, Miss Lisenbe. Oh, and, Sher, please give your grandfather my best. Since he hasn't been at the golf club, I never see him anymore," he added while pushing his cart further toward the checkout area of the food market.

"He acts like Granddad isn't playing golf anymore. That's Granddad's passion," I said watching the rather stately gentleman head happily toward the scanning registers.

"Maybe he's playing somewhere else or with someone else," Kaylee supposed.

"Doubt that. The country club has the best course around here – much better than Larkspur's municipal course. And I don't think he's driving over to Montclair to play, not unless someone invited him to complete a foursome. He's played with the same group of men in Larkspur for as long as I can remember."

"Have you talked with your granddad lately?"

"You know, I guess I haven't." Suddenly I felt selfish, sort of self-absorbed.

"Maybe you should go by and see him, especially since you live in the same town. And you know, since you have a cell phone, it wouldn't be all that hard to at least call him. Now, would it?"

"Kaylee, I ... I just assumed he was staying busy. Just playing golf, fooling around with other seventy-somethings. Doing whatever you do when you're that age," I retorted, unsuccessfully masking my guilt.

I wasn't hungry anymore.

DARDEN NORTH, MD
306

Chapter
20
◆◆◆
THE FOLLOW-THROUGH

My girlfriend wasted no time in arranging my medical training, proving that her rebuttal to Mr. Desselle was not simply drummed-up debate. To my knowledge Kaylee was a truthful woman and meant what she said, did what she meant – definitely one of those types, and I had grown to love her for it. I was surprised, though, to find that she had indeed mentioned my career plans to her doctor in Montclair.

"I'll call Dr. Chamblee's nurse about your following him around for a few days," she said as we departed the market in my car.

"I'm not sure that I'd feel comfortable following a gynie around, and I expect that his patients would feel the same way. You know, the doctor introduces this great-looking, sexy guy to them and says, 'Hi, this is my friend. He wants to be play doctor.' " I laughed alone, suddenly feeling rather adolescent.

Kaylee then looked at me indignantly, as though I truly were childish.

"I hate to put you in your place, young man, but Dr. Chamblee is himself rather good-looking; in fact, he's kinda hot. There's another librarian who goes to him – she's somewhere between forty and fifty, probably closer to fifty. Even she thinks he's hot. But she didn't say he was hot, didn't use that word – said he was sexy, so that puts her more toward fifty, I suppose.

"That's enough, Kaylee. He's a doctor, not a ... "

"Oh, I know. It's just that he's very nice. Several of the girls in my bunko group go to him. We don't fantasize about him or anything like that when we discuss our doctor visits over margaritas – at least I don't." Kaylee hesitated just a tad too long. "I wonder if he dates anyone regularly."

"I think I'd better go with you to your next appointment," I interjected as an answer to what I hoped was a rhetorical question.

Kaylee did not hear me. "He's about six-feet tall, clean-shaven, trim, but with a nice build, probably has a washboard stomach under that scrub suit. But I've never heard him mention anything about that."

"About what?" I asked, growing truly jealous of my girlfriend's doctor but also a little disgusted, more grossed out than anything. "Anyway, how could some guy do what he does all day long and still want to ... "

"Never heard him mention anything about being married or dating anyone; that's what I was talking about. There was some woman in the waiting room a few months ago who was rambling on about Dr. Chamblee, you know about how really cool he was, a hunk without acting like he knew he was one."

"Let's change the subject, or better yet, why don't you change doctors? Pick some geezer somewhere or maybe a lady doctor to go to. Somebody you and your running buddies won't slobber over, unless some of the bunko gals are weird or something."

That suggestion drew no response. Kaylee wasn't really listening to me at that point. Women are like that sometimes. They believe they have a captive audience (or know they do, like when you're in bed with them) and keep the discussions going until some sort of point is made or until you redirect their attention, an action which is generally futile. Men are like that, too, I suppose.

"That reminds me." Kaylee began a renewed rambling discourse, an uncharacteristic trait for her but a topic she found fascinating. "This same waiting room gossip (I don't think she was Dr. Chamblee's patient; I believe she was seeing one of the other doctors) was going on and on about how she had heard that one of the female doctors, the oldest one who practices there, a Dr. Hawes (I think her first name is Aslyn) has been interested in Dr. Chamblee for quite some time."

"Chamblee? The 'Incredible Hunk'?"

Kaylee failed to answer my sarcasm, her train of thought unbroken. "We heard that ol' gossip say ... that is, all the other patients and I heard as we sat together in this little alcove section of the waiting room ... " Kaylee put her forefinger up to her cheek as though playing a detective in an old movie and paused until she remembered the rumormonger's exact chatter. "Let's see," my girlfriend continued, "the woman announced, 'My friend told me that the older woman doctor, that Dr. Hawes, is going through her own midlife crisis by chasing that young, single, male doctor around. Maybe she should put her own self on some of those hormones all the doctors want us to take. Or maybe she has too many hormones already!' " Kaylee added, "Of course, we all laughed and got icy stares from some of the clinic nurses as they whisked by."

"You want me to go over to Montclair on one of my few days off from the fire department and follow those doctors around to get a feel for practicing medicine?" I slipped in edgewise. "Sounds like they're getting a feel for each other; I would agree that those jokers certainly don't need to be taking any extra hormones!" I laughed at length at my observation as Kaylee stared coolly at me, mouth twisted slightly to the right and left eyebrow down turned enough to wrinkle her forehead in the same direction. "Yeah, like the TV show, *Desperate Doctors*," I said, hooting even louder at the purported sleazy antics but remaining solo in the appreciation of my humor.

As Kaylee continued, my laughter trailed off in a death as miserable as that of an audience sitting before a sour late night television comedian. "Yeah, *Hawes*, that's her name. She had a baby less than a year ago, the woman went on to tell us there in the waiting room." Kaylee had not heard any of my one-sided humor as she lowered her voice a few decibels as if in fear that the subject might walk into the waiting room at any minute. "And, you know what, Sher? Dr. Hawes is not even married."

"Kaylee, for gosh sakes, that's really not all that unusual these days, even in Mississippi!"

"But the doctor supposedly didn't even have a boyfriend, at least no one that any of the office staff knew anything about. Even the nurses who work with her all day long had no idea that she was dating anybody."

"How does this woman that you met in that section of the waiting room know all that stuff? Sounds like The Big Mouth just likes to use it."

"No, she explained that she's friends with most of the appointment secretaries and a couple of the clinic nurses."

I hated to admit it, even to myself, but the tale about the horny, middle aged lady doctor who got knocked up was growing more interesting, almost sordid, and indeed would have made a worthwhile episode for a nighttime TV soap.

"She told everybody that she had gotten a sperm donor from an infertility clinic somewhere and had kept the whole thing to herself in case it didn't stick."

"Well, that sounds reasonable. But she's in her forties?"

"You wouldn't know it – looks a whole lot younger. I caught a glimpse of Dr. Hawes one day when she walked through the lab in the clinic. She's a knockout! I wish I knew her secret."

The doctor's secret was probably the result of some colleague's handiwork, I reasoned, but chose not to comment. I did not want to give Kaylee any ideas. I planned a long life with her and from her firm, ample looks believed that she would hold up just fine.

"How did this doctor ... Dr. Hawes ... how did her partners take her news?" I asked, getting interested.

"We all asked the same thing. The woman explained that Dr. Hawes had lost a baby several years back when she was married, so everybody seemed to be really happy for her. Yeah, they were all really happy for her. No questions."

"But Doctor Hunk, I mean *Chamblee*, the one you want me to follow around, he's not supposed to be the sperm donor?"

If I had been writing the episode, I would have made Chamblee the sperm donor; perhaps I'd have him donate between hospital rounds or between breast exams or maybe have him meet the old lady doctor in a dark room where the technicians usually develop x-rays. He would pay the techs to keep quiet, tell them to go out and smoke a cigarette for a few minutes. Then the two lovebirds would put a *HAZARD – DO NOT ENTER* sign on the door, warning others about the dangers inside and turn the film developing machine on full blast. That would muffle all the noise Kaylee's assumed beefcake would create.

The hole in my screenplay was that the medical practice used quiet digital equipment in the x-ray department.

"No, Dr. Chamblee's innocent," Kaylee answered. "The baby doesn't look a thing like him." Before I could question her about the accuracy of her information she explained further, "I asked the woman in the waiting room about that. She said that one of the front office secretaries regularly baby-sits for that lady doctor. The baby's beautiful, well, you know, handsome. It's a little boy after all, but doesn't look a thing like my doctor. "

"Oh, really?"

"Definitely, Sher. The woman told us all that the baby's complexion is a lot darker than Dr. Chamblee's."

Chapter

21

◆◆◆

THE INCISION

To my surprise Kaylee followed through. In less than four
weeks, I was standing in her gynecologist's office, checking in
as instructed with the office manager. The lady's name was Nell
Lowery. Late fiftyish, I decided, and well-preserved, she handed
me a thin stack of forms to complete in longhand, explaining
that the federal government required numerous confidentiality
agreements whenever a student shawdowed one of the doctors or
otherwise worked at the Montclair Center. I reminded her that I
was not a student anymore, not really, that I had graduated from
Ole Miss a few years back and planned to renew my efforts toward
medical school admission.

Mrs. Lowery was polite and encouraging, no doubt the reason
for her longtime employment. "As office manager here, I've been
subjected to many kinds of people. But I can tell that you're one of
the personable types. I'm no clairvoyant, Mr. Foxworth, but I think
you'll get into medical school if you keep at it."

I hoped that this Nell Lowery was correct, at least at the time
I thought I did. My presence in Mrs. Lowery's building was at
my girlfriend's insistence although it was not conditional on her

remaining my girlfriend. I needed someone like Kaylee or maybe
Nell Lowery to look out for me. For the long haul my grandfather
seemed to have given up on his grandson, just as he had his own
existence. Of course, by then my parents had been dead for over
five years, and my view of life had developed into living for the
weekend in the midst of keeping a relationship alive and myself
and my adopted dog fed. To poor old Dickens's detriment, my
primary concern was in keeping that girlfriend happy although the
dog still lived like a king.

"Dr. Chamblee is over at the hospital next door making rounds. I
checked the computer schedule. He had an early surgery, a minor
case, an ETA," Mrs. Lowery explained.

"An ETA? Estimated time of arrival?" I asked while signing
the last in the series of lengthy small-print documents, assuring
anyone who cared that I would not release any information
about anything I saw, heard, felt, or smelled around that medical
office. I remember having a weird feeling about being there in
the first place – a gynecologist's office? Anyway how would this
Dr. Chamblee introduce me to his patients? Or would he even
introduce me to his patients? He certainly was not going to invite
me to get down between the stirrups with him and take a look.
Perhaps he was going to merely stick me in a corner someplace
out of the way and give me some x-rays or a medical journal to
look at. Maybe he would just give me a crossword puzzle to work
and a doughnut to munch on. Maybe they had some crayons and a
coloring book around the joint.

The more I thought about it, the more ridiculous it seemed that
I was even here to observe at the Montclair Center for Women's
Medical and Surgical Services, a gynecologist's office. To avoid
their derision, I had not shared this arrangement with any of my
cohorts at the fire department, even Alvin Coakley. My growing
assumption was that this whole situation was simply a doctor's

polite acquiescence to placate a pretty patient. I believed that Kaylee had probably put Knox Chamblee, MD, in an awkward position, in the professional sense: *make my boyfriend resume his interest in medical school or I'm going to find a new doctor!*

"I'm sure that even though this Chamblee guy is a professional while taking care of women all day, he couldn't be blind or dead," I mumbled as I put down the pen and stood to hand the completed papers to the office manager working at her computer.

"ETA means *endometrial thermal ablation* to us," a male voice explained from inside the door behind me, interrupting my long, chugging train of thought. Startled from reconstructing the circumstances that had placed me in the office, I lost the molded plastic pen I was using, allowing it to bounce along the edge of the office manager's desk. As the writing instrument fell to the floor, I made a spastic and unsuccessful lunge for it.

"Don't worry about it, Mr. Foxworth, please. It's just a freebee from the Ortho rep," Mrs. Lowery reassured me as she retrieved the pen and tossed it more gingerly into a small canister on her desk where others awaited. "Dr. Chamblee, this is the young man you were expecting."

So this is **the** Knox Chamblee, I thought, as I stood straighter and refocused myself, fighting the rush of blood to my cheeks that accompanied the embarrassment over fumbling with the ink pen.

Just as Kaylee had described, the young doctor stood about six feet, maybe even a little taller. However, at first glance he did not meet the real image of a doctor, at least not in my mind, that image being what my plastic surgeon father had presented. Instead of my father's tailored, starched white or light blue shirt consistently adorned with silk tie, Chamblee in contrast donned a surgical scrub suit, the bluish color of which was most likely missing from any known crayon box. His white physician's lab coat was not really wrinkled or really pressed. It was somewhere between clean and dirty – truthfully, closer to clean. Television actors portraying doctors wear such coats along with poorly pressed scrub suits to force a haggard look. But Knox Chamblee, MD, did not appear all that haggard. Since it was early in the day, he probably had not had enough time to get that way.

"Hi, I'm Knox Chamblee and you're ... "

"Sheridan Foxworth." I was not sure why I used my complete name at that moment because I haven't been called Sheridan since – well, I can't remember when. Maybe I needed the few extra letters included in my surname to make up for the *MD* missing from the *Foxworth*.

"Oh, yes, I've been looking forward to having you here and showing you around, Sheridan."

"Uh, call me *Sher*."

"Well, sure, now that you mention it, that's how Kaylee referred to you. And you can call me ... " My anal sphincter tightened, dreading the requirement to call him *Dr. Chamblee*, since he really did not appear much my senior " ... call me *Knox*." The guy really was not pompous, not at all. But neither was my dad, although he was better dressed than Chamblee.

"Endometrial thermal ablation is a technique we have to treat patients who are having really bad menstrual periods," Chamblee continued, "as an alternative to major surgery and when medication has not helped to control the excessive monthly bleeding. It's fairly new on the scene but is showing itself in some cases to be useful as an alternative to hysterectomy."

"Uh, do you do a lot of surgery?" I really did not know what to ask or say and then suddenly remembered that I had not thanked Chamblee at all for having me out to his office. After I did so, he walked us from Nell Lowery's office, and I followed as if a medical student trailing a great professor.

"Sure, we're happy to have you out here. We'll let you see what we do all day out in the world of ob/gyn. The day can be fairly unpredictable as you might imagine, but, yes, we do perform a fair amount of surgery in between delivering babies, lots of babies." Chamblee grinned happily as he mentioned the babies, gesturing with hands spread widely apart as though describing the big catch. Through this enthusiastic display, he seemed to find great power and satisfaction in his part toward expanding the planet's population.

"On the other end of the spectrum, I've got a hysterectomy to do at noon today, between the morning and afternoon clinics. You can observe and even dress out in the OR if you like. I'll just have to ask the patient if it's all right with her and then fill out a few OSHA and other confidentiality forms."

"No, I think I might just sit on the bench and watch," I answered lightheartedly, but he seemed to miss the comparison. As I followed alongside him, uncertain of where we were headed within the building, Chamblee's body movements and mannerisms reflected those of someone who did not miss a thing, a mind constantly in gear, thinking and moving ahead.

"Have you had much experience scrubbing in surgery?" he asked as we rounded the next corner, passing a section of tall interior plants whose well-manicured leaves glimmered with polish in the rays falling from the skylight above.

"Not unless you can call dissecting a fetal pig or a stiff cat in biology classes at Ole Miss a type of surgery," I answered. Once more, the levity was lost.

"You see, our field of medicine has a good mix of medical and surgical care. A whole lot of stuff can go on during the day and night around here: deliveries, ectopic pregnancies, miscarriages, diagnosis of cancerous and non-cancerous tumors, treatment of STDs, dealing with patients' marital problems ... you name it." Again Chamblee spread his arms wide like the fisherman as we rounded another corner and entered an area containing flat computer screens and smooth Formica-covered desktop spaces.

A diminutive African-American woman, whose name I would soon learn was Lovejoy, was sitting in front of a mound of papers and folders stacked in the first cubicle, shuffling them into separate stacks. I sensed that deep-down she was kind and friendly. "I thought that computer system upgrade was supposed to get rid of most of this stuff," she said as though talking to herself but directing the remark to her boss, who was leading me in her direction. After the introductions, Lovejoy Montez suggested that I sit in a chair nearby while she prepared the first patient visit for Dr. Chamblee.

When he walked away for a moment she surprised me. "You seem like a nice boy, Sher, but let me tell you something. I've been Dr. Chamblee's office nurse ever since he started here, and if the good Lord will somehow let you turn out to be just like him, you'll make a mighty good doctor."

"You see, Miss Montez, this whole thing was my girlfriend's idea and for two reasons: number one, she wants to seal the commitment, on my part, that is, not hers – hers is already sealed airtight, real airtight – to my becoming a doctor and number two, she believes my hanging around some real doctors in all this will add weight to my med school application." As the disclaimer defining my intentions was completed, I found myself waving my arms around as though encompassing all of the surroundings in my reference to *this*: soaking in every computer terminal, fluffy couch, clipboard, blood pressure cuff, and passerby. The arm motions were not deliberate; they were reflexive but at the same time almost hesitant, reaching for something that might be truly unreachable for me.

Was *this* whole thing possible for Sheridan Foxworth III? Even though his was a different generation, my father had made it to and through med school and then successfully survived brutal general surgery and plastic surgery residencies. And was he smarter or more talented than I? I'm certain he did not screw up his freshman year in college as I did, but then he wasn't carting around the same heavy emotional baggage. Growing up, I had never asked Dad specifics about his university GPA or the height of his MCAT scores. To do such a nerdy thing had never occurred to me. Likewise, why would he ever offer such information?

Quickly my self-dissection was interrupted. "First, Son, for whatever reason you're here, don't call me *Mrs. Montez*. For Pete's sake, call me *Lovejoy*. Also around this office you'll need to do whatever I tell you to do and with no smart mouth, and we'll get along just fine, just fine and dandy."

"Yes, ma'am," I replied almost in salute.

"Drop the *ma'am*, too, Sugga, 'cause I sure don't look like your mother and if you're thinkin' of your grandmother, I should pop you. I'm way the wrong color anyway. And, besides, we don't need to get anywhere near that ol' *mammy* stuff. We're all way past that, way past it."

Almost embarrassed, I laughed a little at her rambling response and token reference to racial equality issues. My laughter was in acceptance of what I sensed as a true offer of friendship, an invitation that was silently but readily accepted. I ascertained correctly that Lovejoy Montez was one of those people that you simply wanted on your side, the kind that would do anything within reason to help you, even without your asking.

"Now, why don't you sit down in this chair over here out of my way and the doctor's way for just a few minutes and let the two of us get organized for the morning appointments. Dr. Chamblee stayed much too long over at the hospital. After he completed his surgery case, he probably stopped by to say hello to that pretty social worker over there. She's been running after him for about

a year and I 'spect has caught up with him by now, most likely
several times and on a regular basis, I would imagine."

A near guttural laugh trailed the air behind her as Lovejoy
walked away, then rapidly exploded into a cackle of infinite
self-pleasure over the metaphor. As the assistant to Dr. Knox
Chamblee rounded the corner and moved back to the main patient
waiting area, I looked forward to this rare opportunity to enter
the shameless arena of Larkspurian hearsay – a chance to tell
my sweet, gorgeous girlfriend something that she did not already
know. A quick cell phone call to Kaylee with details regarding the
private life of her precious Knox Chamblee would blow her away.

"Hey, Baby, guess what your wonderful Dr. Chamblee does
between rounds at the hospital?" I plotted to tell her, expecting
a response like *what are you talking about, Sher?* "He's making
some in-and-outs, too!" I would tell her before her denials of
such improprieties. The details might need to be spiced up a
bit, though, I thought, just to get more of a rise out of Kaylee.
However, revealing Lovejoy's abstract information about the social
worker that the doctor was dating would be no less enthralling
to my own girlfriend than something juicier. She would realize
that outside the examination room Chamblee led a more realistic
private life than she and her peers had fantasized about: he
liked girls closer to his own age. Nevertheless, Kaylee and her
Bunko friends would be engrossed with even the tiniest personal
revelation about Knox Chamblee, MD, and be shocked by my
trumping them. I looked forward to making that call.

Meanwhile, things remained quiet where Lovejoy had assigned
me to sit at attention and await further instructions. My mind
had begun to race, partly out of boredom and partly from
nervous anticipation of what was next. Nearby I spotted a folded
newspaper but did not dare reach for it. What kind of impression
would that make, I wondered. Knox Chamblee would dart up

to tell me about some sort of one-of-a kind medical finding, a fascinoma, and there I'd be sitting – a lazy dumbass reading the newspaper, somebody who'd never get into medical school, but instead is destined to rot around a fire pole.

Hastily I decided to slip Kaylee a text message on my cell phone. The note about Chamblee's love life would arrive to her in-box simultaneous with the opening of the Larkspur Public Library for the day. Her stories continued to amaze me, those of discovering patrons anxiously waiting in line at the front door when she unlocked it from the inside.

Unlike most other southern women, Kaylee generally kept her cell phone attached to her body in some fashion, not buried deep in a purse waiting for a frantic scramble to quiet a chirping ring, loud buzz, or downloaded theme song. Today she had it in the pocket of a linen jacket and responded promptly to my sent message. The resulting exchange progressed into bantering, back-and-forth texting as I kept a watchful eye for anyone approaching. Kaylee's reaction to my Knox Chamblee news bulletin had been as I had expected. Despite her immediate and seemingly desperate request for more specific information about the hospital social worker, I flatly refused Kaylee's request that I find my way over to the hospital next door to check out the girl.

Around the corner from where I was busy thumb-typing was a patient waiting area that served as a stopping point before an audience with the doctor. On the edge of this well-appointed space rested a comfortable-looking upholstered piece of furniture, a loveseat of sorts, filled with a man and woman engaged in deep conversation. I immediately recognized him as Minor Leblanc. They were a curiously incongruous couple, but as they remained entirely focused on one another, I persisted with typing away in a clandestine electronic discussion with my girlfriend.

"You know, Miz Madelyn, I noticed a couple of the doctors, a man and a lady doctor, talking to the secretaries when we walked in the front of this office. Neither of them had on a suit, not even a tie or a nice silk blouse. I think that's horrid! If a doctor's got to tell me that I've got cancer or something awful like that, I want the guy to look nice," he said to Madelyn Gwinn in an effort to lighten the moment. Although she smiled politely at his humorous attempt, Minor Leblanc sensed her persistent uneasiness with life.

"Keep your lips on," he continued. "Everything will be great. Trust me."

"Oh, Minor, I'm really not sure."

"You can wear that wonderful leather jacket that we got for you in Chicago last year. It still looks perfect. Fabulous! Fabulous!" This plan was followed by a few discomfited moments of silence as Minor Leblanc felt more than awkward in mentioning that now infamous shopping trip. Although serving then as a paid consulting stylist, he fell in the role of a true friend when he had had to break the news to Madelyn regarding her husband's untimely death.

One of Minor Leblanc's most productive clients, Madelyn Gwinn had indeed had a difficult last year. Her husband was killed, and she had undergone brain surgery, albeit successful – certainly enough of a struggle for even the most stoic of individuals. "Minor, but this thing that the Larkspur school is putting on is so important. Cullen (she paused a moment, lowering her head slightly below the horizon in reverence to her late physician husband) was so interested in all of the area schools, not only the ones in Montclair, like this Larkspur Something-or-Other school. I'm not sure what they are calling that private academy now. Anyway, he delivered so many babies through the years and had so many patients come to see him from all around this area that I know he would have said *Yes* to helping sponsor the fundraiser – even though it's going to be at the home of those – those people.

"Now, Miz Madelyn, this party at the Pixlers is going to be fabulous. They are a lovely couple, and you yourself are going to look so absolutely gorgeous that night," Minor reassured her with complete sincerity.

"Oh, Minor. I just don't know. I just … "

"Look out, Mad! You're on your way back, forever!" Leblanc exclaimed as though the two were the only ones around, his hands lifted in the air as if in praise. "Everyone will believe that you've had more done to you this year than just brain surgery. Just let me look at you: your face, your hair, your physique – it all just screams youth. Oh, Jesus. It just screams youth! We just need to work a little on the gear."

Mrs. Cullen Gwinn smiled politely at Minor Leblanc on whom she continued to rely as a personal shopper, grooming advisor, friend, and more recently as escort on such seemingly mundane errands. Recuperating from the emotional and physical trauma of the last many months had made even appearing in public among her peers an exhausting challenge, although lately she had begun to regain her stamina and self-confidence.

"Minor, you were so thoughtful to come with me to the doctor today," Madelyn whispered kindly. "I needed to get in here for a check-up because I can't neglect my health, you know. Cullen would not have been able to stand it, letting myself go and all."

"Now, Miz Gwinn, you know that we can both hear Doc saying, 'My sweet, Mad, my fabulous wife, you've got to carry on without me. You can do it. You go ahead and let our friend Minor help you.' "

Since Madelyn Gwinn had recovered from surgery to repair a cerebral aneurysm, her headaches had ceased, although a block of memory had not returned. Her head was physically healed and the lovely hair grown back, but there remained bits and pieces of her life that were more than cloudy. She had gradually resumed a busy social life in Montclair and surrounding communities, initially appearing frail to those who cared. But now, her stamina and interest in life were rejuvenating. No longer the matriarch of a medical dynasty, she had instead settled into the role of widow of a well-respected area physician.

Her upcoming early morning appointment that day was with a young doctor, Knox Chamblee, MD. Appropriately, Chamblee had been her late husband's hand-picked hire to join the medical clinic he had founded many years before. While Minor Leblanc did not customarily provide escort to physicians' offices, he had sensed his treasured client's uneasiness about returning there. Besides, he was anxious to get Madelyn Gwinn's outfit selection finalized for the fundraiser at the Pixler Estate. After giving her first dibs on many of his recent design finds, he needed to move on toward completing the same for other billable customers.

And he knew that he would have a captive audience with Mrs. Gwinn during the drive over and wait to see the doctor. Doctors always kept people waiting.

"Miz Madelyn, we're going to have you looking really hot at that party."

"Minor, I haven't looked *hot* in thirty years!"

"Nonsense. We'll do that wonderful leather jacket over this inviting black criss-cross top I've got on hold for you in Dallas and team it with a black pant highlighted with these adorable pockets. You'll barely be able to see them peeking out from under the bottom of the jacket. The effect will be more than anyone will be able to stand, particularly your date."

"Minor, I'm not sure I'm going to go with a date."

"You just must," he emphasized with eyes wide and mouth drawn in concern. "Don't turn that man down!"

"Well, I was going to the thing anyway when he called and had even bought my ticket." Madelyn looked out toward the window on the far wall. "Cullen would have wanted me to go to the fundraiser," she repeated. "But I just don't feel right about going out with a man yet; it's oh-so-soon."

"Miz Madelyn, Doc would want you to move on with your life. I know he would. At first I tossed and turned in my bed the other night when you called me about the invitation. Then suddenly Jesus told me I should encourage you to go. Doc is in heaven pushing you on. You are his beautiful wife, but he's gone now, and he wants you to be happy here on this earth. Jesus told me so."

Madelyn focused on Minor's eyes, which appeared steady, serious, and truthful. He was a good friend, the best.

"But I told Tricia Pennington about going with a date, maybe even just calling it an escort. She told me not to go with him, that everyone would whisper at the party about my being out with another man. You know, saying that it's too soon and all after Cullen's death."

"Is that for real? It can't be! That's the tackiest thing I've ever heard," he retorted in a voice inflection that startled Madelyn and a woman nearby who was deep into a magazine article on Tom Cruise. Before ditching him for a stylist competitor based out of Jackson, Tricia Pennington had been a demanding, former client of Minor Leblanc. "You're ready to carry on with your life, and nobody will think for a single minute that a fine woman like you will be carrying on with that gentleman." Minor glanced away for a few seconds before turning back. "It's just an outing, anyway, I would think.

"Anyway, my dear Miz Madelyn. You're going to be fabulous forever in this outfit I'm – we're – putting together for that night. It's you forever! Nobody at the big house party will be thinking about him anyway. They won't even see him in the rays bouncing off you. They'll be blinded by your radiance."

"Oh, Minor!" Madelyn laughed as he appealed to the vanity that she could no longer keep in check.

"We'll put on those long diamond and gold ears, the ones I brought over to you a couple of nights ago and then add that emerald bracelet I found for you last week."

"But what about shoes? I've got those black ... "

"No, not those things," he interrupted with a distasteful stare. "For sure we must remember our elevation, and even though shoes are at the bottom, they can really put you on your way. But not to worry your sweet little head, or toes, Miz Madelyn. Tonight I'm going to bring over this killer pair of Stuart Weitzman anklestrap shoes with the closed toe. Yes, toooo-diiieee-foooorrrr! But you might have to take them off to dance, depending on how wild you get that night on the Pixlers' patio."

"Oh, Minor!" Madelyn burst into an even more exuberant laugh that once again caught the attention of the now-annoyed magazine reader. She had moved on to an engrossing article about Hollywood pregnancies and the stylish way to give birth in Beverly Hills.

"Sher." Lovejoy had walked up behind me as I had pressed *Send* in response to Kaylee's last text message response. Obviously startled at the interruption, it is possible that I might have even let out a little yelp of guilt, although I really do not remember. "Dr. Chamblee has a patient in the treatment room who gave us permission to let you in to observe. We sort of told her you were already a medical student – told her your name was Extern Foxworth, but that you would have the title of *Intern* one day soon."

I followed Lovejoy down the short hall as I folded the cell phone back to credit card configuration and slid it into my lower right coat pocket. She had outfitted me with a short white lab jacket so that I would blend into the surroundings. "Oh, and put that thing on *Silent*, or better yet turn the damn thing off. Didn't you see the *NO CELL PHONE USE PLEASE* sign in the front?" she asked in a tone that was somewhere beneath that of admonishment, more toward disparaging humor. "That notice is really for the patients because all of us employees keep a cell phone handy. The doctors do it, too. We're normal people just like everybody else; we just don't let the things ring." Lovejoy added with amusement, "The doctors hate it when they're doing someone's breast or pelvic exam and the patient reaches over to answer her silly cell phone."

I followed Lovejoy to a thick metal door crafted to resemble a paneled wood one, labeled *Procedure Room*. Underneath this was additional labeling covered with a sliding section of black plastic. As we walked into the room unannounced, although we were certainly expected, Lovejoy quickly slid the cover to the right as an afterthought, exposing the words *In Use*.

The patient was sitting at the edge of an examination table, half unclothed or half dressed, depending on one's perspective. Chamblee was sitting directly in front of her on a rolling stool, holding a diminutive laptop used to record medical information.

"Oh, good. Here's Lovejoy. Now we can go ahead and see what's going on here. Oh, and, Charlotte," he said, referring to his patient, who appeared to be an extremely worried, middle-aged Caucasian with a slight tremor induced by her current situation, "this is the medical student we told you about, Extern Foxworth." Charlotte turned her head enough to nod in awareness at both Lovejoy and the extern but her eyes saw nothing. While I certainly did not recognize this Charlotte, I wondered for a moment about her. To me she resembled a schoolteacher or maybe a bank teller, but for all I knew she could have been a lawyer, doctor, or even an astronaut. In such an humbling position in a doctor's office, one's occupation is certainly irrelevant.

Lovejoy assisted the nervous woman in lying down while securing her feet in metal holders at the end of the table. "Now, Baby, you just put your feet in these stirrups and relax so the doctor can see," she coaxed successfully. Although Charlotte was now properly positioned for Chamblee's examination and remained silent, her reluctance to proceed was evident. While Charlotte's goal was to remain cooperative, my challenge was to keep a stone cold facial expression, a difficult task while imagining Chamblee's head in the female patient's reflexive leg lock. Later I wanted to ask Lovejoy or Knox Chamblee if that had ever happened, but I didn't.

"Now, we're going to take a look here to see what's causing you all this pain," Dr. Chamblee said in a coaxing, gentle voice that failed to soothe his patient's nerves.

As I watched his face from inside the closed door, he showed no apparent surprise in what he saw. "Charlotte, you have a small, thrombosed hemorrhoid that needs to be lanced."

"Well, it certainly doesn't feel small!" Charlotte almost yelled in retort, then restrained her voice. "And it sure didn't look very small either, particularly when I got down with a mirror and looked at it. I tossed and turned all night with the pain. I just know I've got cancer!" she blurted more loudly as she clutched the thin white paper covering the examination table and ripped off a wad.

As though on an automatic cue, Lovejoy moved closer to the now terrified patient, taking her left hand in compassionate support. Charlotte then reached with her right over her body toward Lovejoy to cover the top of the nurse's reassuring hand. Somehow the miserable patient kept her legs still in cooperation.

"Now, Charlotte, this problem here has no typical appearance of cancer." I wondered why he didn't just come out and announce, "You don't have cancer, Charlotte; I promise," but as I have learned since, physicians just do not offer guarantees. "We've shrunk your hemorrhoids before with medication," Chamblee continued calmly, "and this one does resemble a typical hemorrhoid except it has a little hard blood clot in it and meds won't shrink it. It's what we call *thrombosed*, and if it were any larger, I'd have to send you to a general surgeon to take care of it. But since we've caught it in time, I can handle it for you."

"Dr. Chamblee, you've just told me I have a blood clot!" Charlotte strained her head upward and forward staring at her doctor in horror. "Blood clots go to your lungs and kill you quick. I know because I had a cousin that ... "

"No, no, no, it's not that kind of blood clot," he forced reassurance while hiding a tinge of annoyance over the ignorance of this educated patient. As he continued a beefed-up effort toward patient education, Lovejoy worked to release Charlotte's tightening grip on her right hand which was acquiring a bluish cast despite her own dark skin. "A hemorrhoid is a type of vein in the rectal area that doesn't function properly and lets blood sort of stagnate in its passageway. Inflammation and swelling set in, and then there's a lot of pain."

"Right, tell me about it," she interrupted, actually showing a hint of humor as she relaxed her grip on Lovejoy. Nevertheless, the patient's levity was brief as her body tremor returned to dramatically worsen in silence.

In rote fashion, Lovejoy pried her fingers away from the crippling grasp and withdrew a printed paper form from a nearby cabinet in the room. After scribbling on it with a black pen she had pulled from her jacket pocket, she almost whispered, "Baby, just sign this short form for me so we'll have permission to take care of this little hemorrhoid problem for you."

"Aren't you gonna deaden it first?" resumed a strained, shaky voice from the upper end of the exam table that seemed a mark of surrender. The trembling inquiry coordinated with the rest of the body's quiver.

"Sure, of course we are. This hemorrhoid problem is really too minor to ... "

"Minor? Maybe for you it's minor, but not for me, Dr. Chamblee!" Charlotte retorted with renewed strength while attempting to lift her head to a better angle between her spread knees, her stare at the doctor a piercing glare. The exhausting effort was unsuccessful and she sank back on the pillow at the head of the exam table.

"Charlotte, by *minor* I mean *small*. We could take you to the hospital operating room to do this office surgery but generally something like this is done quickly under local anesthesia."

"Okay, go ahead. I'm sorry I'm getting so worked up over this – I really don't know why. I definitely don't want you to do it in the hospital because I'm deathly afraid of being put to sleep."
The anxious patient then acquiesced and signed the office consent form for the recommended incision and evacuation procedure. "Please, please help me, Dr. Chamblee. I just want it to stop hurting."

"That's exactly what we're going to do, Charlotte. Let's go ahead and take care of this for you," he advised sympathetically although I detected a sly eye roll directed toward Lovejoy. Likewise, I almost grinned, surprising myself and hiding the indiscretion by covering my mouth as though a yawn. "First, I'm going to inject one percent lidocaine with epinephrine right where we need it."
As Chamblee explained in detail the process of administering local anesthesia to deaden the area, Lovejoy assembled the supplies for the procedure, displaying them quietly on the cabinet surface adjacent to the examination table.

"Now, how did you say you were going to deaden me, Dr. Chamblee?"

"Uhh, with a needle, a very short, thin one," he answered with indetectable forced patience, beginning to wonder just how really

confused poor Charlotte was over the treatment of her ordeal.
"The effect of the lidocaine will be quick, and then we'll open the
hemorrhoid right at the worst spot to remove the ... " (he stopped
himself before repeating *clot* and used the more universal word
problem) " ... problem giving you almost immediate relief."

Charlotte lay silent, nodding her head weakly in acceptance of
her fate and physically reaffirming her consent to the procedure.

"After we take care of the ... problem, we'll pack the area with a
little piece of gauze and let it remain in place for a few days."

"What will I have to do then?" her voice much weaker, much
more pathetic.

"You'll need to soak in the tub frequently and do something we
call a hot sitz bath. That will really make it feel good. Of course, I'll
send you home with a prescription for some cream to put on the
area."

"Well, I want some pain pills, too! And something stronger than
Darvocet," Charlotte came alive again with an exasperated tone,
still fighting to control her need to quiver. Despite the difficult
patient's outburst, Knox was pleased that she at least seemed to
demonstrate improved comprehension. Working to end their
joint predicament, he injected the lidocaine into and around the
thrombosed area with a thin needle, as promised, borrowed from a
diminutive tuberculin syringe.

"Dr. Chamblee, it you don't quit hurting me, I'm going to use
the *F* word!" Charlotte warned. However, out of necessity her
doctor pushed on with the painful anesthetic injection as she gave
up and stared at the ceiling. The swollen, inflamed anal vein had,
of course, tortured the poor patient to the fullest, that torment
openly shared with the three of us surrounding her in the room.
The remainder of the procedure, which had lengthened from a
scheduled ten minutes to a one hour ordeal for everyone, was
completed successfully and with great satisfaction to Charlotte.

Fortunately, she experienced less discomfort during the incision and evacuation of the blood clot itself than she had revealed during the preoperative examination or in the administration of the local anesthesia. The patient's relief was shared by all, including Extern Foxworth, as the healthcare providers and patient exchanged thank-yous once everything was finally over.

As Charlotte left Chamblee's area of the office, seemingly happy and relieved, and moved toward the check-out area of the clinic, Lovejoy handed her a list of patient instructions that she would probably never read, a prescription for acetaminophen with hydrocodone to use once the local wore off, and a bill.

Watching his patient round the corner out of hearing range, Knox Chamblee asked me, "Still want to go to medical school? Well, get ready; 'cause that was nothin'."

Chapter
22

• • •

THE PARTY HAPPY

The checkout girl scanned Wayne's first item after he placed it on the conveyer belt, and it rolled within easy reach. There was no employee-customer eye contact, and that was all right with Simmons. A professional in his line of work needed to remain anonymous, nondescript. To appear uneasy while making a simple purchase at a discount store would have been a violation of that dogma. Like any other criminal, he never expected to be caught; he was too good, too smooth – and like any other criminal, he never thought of himself as one.

Indeed, Wayne kept his cool when accumulating supplies just as he did when he worked a job. He knew surveillance cameras were mounted in the ceilings and over passageways, probably more than could be detected if one were actually probing for them. Those cameras were probably activated now, recording every angle of his face, every subtle move. Somehow the inevitability of being immortalized on those dim, grainy videos was exciting to Wayne Simmons even though he never planned for any law enforcement officer to study them on his behalf.

His cart overflowed with Wal-Mart's remaining stock of Party

Happy candles, now rumored to be headed for manufacturer's recall if one believed the *Consumer Reveals* website. Wayne knew what the candles were capable of doing, and they had performed splendidly for him on several other jobs. The decorative objects, although that description was certainly subjective, came in assorted colors and consisted of dyed oil floating in and filling clear, thin glass containers. The breakable vessels were then supported by twisted metal frames, painted to match the oil.

During a previous walk through that local Wal-Mart was actually when he had first spotted the Party Happy candles. Sometimes he visited a site one or two months ahead of time to size things up as he had in this case, principally when he was commissioned well in advance and the project was a big one. No question about it, the upcoming one in Larkspur would be sizable.

Larkspur in his opinion had always been a crummy town, and during that site visit he had found nothing changed: a crummy town with a Wal-Mart, a crummy town filled with overly-large, austere houses. But to Wayne Simmons the Wal-Mart was the antithesis to those ostentatious buildings, an extremely hospitable commercial establishment, a virtual wonderland filled with creative possibilities. Not only was there a vast grocery department connected to the housewares section, there was also an optometrist and booming pharmacy that carried everything from low-carbohydrate candy to multicolored, flavored condoms.

As he passed by the checkout area across the front interior of the building, he dodged what he thought might be a camouflaged surveillance camera by ducking into the optometrist's booth. The large printed poster displayed on a metal stand near the alcove's entrance professed that Dr. Wiley O'Neill was an independent doctor of optometry, whatever that meant. Remembering that a great deal of time had elapsed since another doctor had advised him to have his vision rechecked, he considered slipping into the optometrist's booth for a quick, on-demand eye exam. After all, that's what the poster offered in smaller bold print: NO WAITING, NO APPOINTMENT NECESSARY.

When a fire ignition source erupted prematurely during a different engagement, his ocular orbits had been nearly flash-dried. His not losing total eyesight had been a miracle, according to the doctor he slipped in to see afterward, and it had been much too long since he was to re-appoint for another eye exam. The temptation to take care of himself was natural to self-preservation, but he worried about a lengthy session in that Wal-Mart examinee chair, especially if a surveillance camera was mounted somewhere in the ceiling tiles above. In addition, he doubted if there were many requirements of patient confidentiality in a medical facility crammed into a discount store. Bringing too much attention to someone who needed to remain nondescript, essentially faceless, was too much of a risk for Wayne Simmons. So there in Wal-Mart he nixed the impulse to protect his health, at least for then. Besides, he realized that hanging around places like a busy store to purchase supplies was risky enough.

Simmons moved away from the optometrist department, sliding toward the bowels of the store. There were people everywhere, fondling merchandise endorsed by various entertainment celebrities. "Buying crap they don't need," he said to himself. "Rich people are just like these blue-collars, only they wouldn't be caught dead in a ... " Simmons' judgmental murmurings halted as he was drawn to them. There they were – the answer – the merchandise he required – candles, but not just any candles. "Holy, shit! Why hadn't I already figured this out? Damn!"

A woman who was choosing her flavor of Diet Coke from the cases stacked nearby looked at him with disapproving surprise, then resumed with a selection of the cherry vanilla variety. She had passed over his items of interest, considering them gaudy, tasteless, tacky. Those very attributes of design were the sordid allure for Wayne Simmons, master artist of arson. The boxes and cartons of Party Happy candles were doing more than simply gathering dust in the section adjacent to the stacks of Coke Zero, Coke, Diet Coke, Cherry Diet Coke, Black Cherry Vanilla Diet Coke, Vanilla Diet Coke, and Lime Diet Coke along with the decaffeinated and alternative sweetener varieties. The colorful glass and metal oil candles were screaming for his attention. Suddenly Wayne no longer felt the desire or need to have his eyes examined; his vision was perfectly clear. "Those eye doctors can go to hell," his remorseless inflection again almost loud enough for the woman by him to hear. In seeing the real value of an object, at least from the perspective of his line of work, he believed his eyesight to be entirely accurate, definitely much better than that of most people.

"You know what they say about another man's trash," he intoned, lowering his voice to a whisper while wiping away the layer of dust atop the Party Happy boxes. The store's inventory displayed all three available shapes and several colors made possible by the flammable metallic paint intended to coordinate with every décor, no matter how tasteless. The woman addicted to various flavors of Diet Coke did not hear Wayne as she hurriedly pushed away with a weighted cart containing three of her favorite cases, none caffeine free.

Since the product recall was future news, the store still had an ample inventory including all available candle shapes: rectangular, square, and oblong, each meant to be decorative to someone. Wayne had long ago decided that he had something of a flair for that sort of thing.

As he selected the packed carton from the top of the stack, blowing the last bit of dust into the next aisle, he decided quietly, "I might just have to keep one of these jewels for myself." Wayne gently picked a boxed unit out of the full carton which he had carefully secured inside his own shopping cart. As though handling a newborn, raising it to eye-level and scrutinizing it through the cellophane viewing windows, he judged, "Might look nice in my living room. That is, if I had a living room." Wayne could barely contain his delight as he filled the cart with as many boxes of the unassembled candle units as possible without causing breakage and quickly headed to the checkout.

Generally Wayne liked to research the potential value of an addition to his arsenal, particularly regarding its efficiency as a source of combustion. In spite of his certainty that the Party Happy would do the job well, he planned to reassure himself just in case. An internet search of the product and its manufacturer was the first step to that process. Since the motels frequented by Simmons were not the type to provide internet services, free or otherwise, and the one in Larkspur was no exception, he utilized the public library for his electronic research. Wayne had also begun to realize that this venue might be less traceable than a motel room, even one paid for in cash. Happily, Wayne had noticed that the Larkspur Public Library was convenient to the Wal-Mart, allowing him to walk the few blocks carrying his new treasures in two large shopping bags. Alternately he had considered rolling off with his purchases stuffed into a stolen shopping cart but did not want to be thought homeless or be chased by store security. As he trodded along the sidewalk toward the library, Wayne glanced up to catch the Diet Coke woman speeding by in a grey Suburban; she was obviously watching him through her rearview mirror.

The public library was situated on a short side street, leading off the main drag from Wal-Mart, and nestled among tall, mature trees and other established vegetation as though the building also grew there. The architecture was such that Simmons felt unsure of the structure's actual age, a potential problem in his line of work but not a concern since Wayne had no intention of torching the library. The library's street was quiet and restful, and Wayne liked that. Everything about a library was supposed to be quiet.

A pretty librarian whose name badge read *Miss Lisenbe* helped him with the computer although he really required no help, but he had spotted her across the room and wanted to be closer to her, even if only for a moment. The Theories Manufacturing website gave no hint about the impending product recall that the company was indeed quietly fighting. For the reasons that Wayne Simmons had recognized in advance of the company engineers, each Party Happy unit would provide an extremely efficient ignition source, particularly when employed in groups.

Wayne had already deciphered what the consumer watchdog groups expected and would eventually prove in demanding a recall of the decorative fixtures: the metallic paint sprayed on the composite metal frame supporting the oil-filled glass was highly flammable, perfect for his purposes. Once the candle was lit and the oil heated, the paint covering the metal would ignite in only a few minutes. The glass would shatter in an explosion of scorching oil that would spray anything within a radius of three linear feet. Considering the circular pattern of the blast, the fiery spectacle of oil, glass, and colored smoke would actually encompass an area of nearly thirty feet squared.

His last science class at what had become the Larkspur Institute for Education had been a treasure trove of knowledge at least for one student, at least pertaining to the information that Wayne Simmons deemed important and interesting. The text's chapter on combustion and kinetics had included a multi-page treatise on candles, a chapter which had been glossed over by the bored Gregory Whitestone but which still fascinated Wayne, his student. Simmons read and reread the illustrated paragraphs to near memorization and could still recite the chapter's summarizing paragraph: *A simple beeswax candle crowned by a laminar flame creates only fifty watts of heat as the flame emits a temperature approaching 900 degrees centigrade, hot by any standard, yet the outer combustion zone can radiate a temperature as high as 1400 centigrade. Metal in close proximity could melt, particularly if the metal does not remove the heat or scatter the heat in any sort of a safe dilution pattern.*

If only the supervising engineer of the candle company, who was fired well before the firm's bankruptcy petition, had understand that dictum. The misconception of basic science principles portrayed by the Theodis Candle Manufacturing Company had resulted in the eventual doom of their darling product, the Party Happy decorative candle, as well as of the inventions that followed.

The carelessness of the Party Happy candle's blueprint did not cease with the combustible paint or the hazardous metal. In an effort to accentuate the color of the aromatic oils topping off the glass containers, the designer provided for multiple wicks to emanate a brighter light. Hence, here was evidence of another flaw clearly learned from that chemistry class: *the wax or other combustible material encasing the wick or wicks of a candle must liquefy at such a rate as to expose just enough wick to keep the candle lit.* One might think (if one thinks of such things, but Wayne Simmons spent most of his waking hours thinking of such things) of a candle's fuel being the wax or oil or whatever comprises the body of the candle. But the source of the light is the candle's wick – not a difficult concept to grasp. If the candle flame is not provided with a steady supply of fresh wick to burn, then the exposed wick burns to a thin cinder and sputters out quietly. During this process of providing illumination, the wax or oil supporting the burning wick becomes sootless carbon dioxide and water if the laminar flame is smooth. If there is too much wick material available to burn, then, of course, the candle will emit an excessive amount of heat, especially if the wick is not centered within the body of the candle itself. That temperature extreme contained within a limited space would transform the flawed Party Happy candle into a potential fire bomb as the scorching aromatic oil torched its highly flammable painted metal casing.

Wayne's internet research had taken him to information outlining the aftermath of the candle's faulty design, thereby cinching his plan. Several Party Happies had accidentally been left burning overnight in an Atlanta spa by a frustrated masseuse kept overtime by a demanding client. The mistake could not have created a better fire. Lots and lots of Party Happies were left happily burning and scattered within an inviting décor of thick, fluffy, dry bath towels. The result was the torching of an entire shopping center. Not long after Wayne Simmons would finish using his stash, that careless incident would actually propel the product recall movement. At any rate, the Larkspur Wal-Mart would have none to pack for return. Its supply had been stripped by Simmons.

Long before consumer advocate groups, the high school-level scientist in Wayne Simmons delightfully discovered another facet of the flawed candle. The Party Happy, the flagship product of the Theodis Candle Manufacturing Company, could and would under many conditions reignite spontaneously upon being extinguished. His secret discovery became a backup plan should anyone snuff out his little jewels prematurely.

Wayne was exuberant, believing his research had culminated in the ideal ignition source for the Pixler project. "Yeah, these babies oughta torch everyone of those high-priced curtains, or draperies, or whatever you call 'em. I bet they'll have a lot of big, overstuffed furniture pushed up real close against them curtains. Nope, it won't take long. That place'll be gone in no time. There'll be so much screamin' and yellin'! Women and men both – they'll be shitless!" Despite his private school education, Wayne's slaughter of the English language was just that: a vernacular that would horrify any English teacher, most preachers, and the scholarship donors who had paid for that education.

Wayne was right on track. Once he had learned of the candles and compiled his *modus operandi*, all he needed was inside access to the site. The colossal preparations surrounding the institute's fundraiser were providing just that. As the school board president had predicted during his lobbying of Rachel Pixler, several catering agencies fell over themselves seeking involvement. Since the businesses were in such dire need of manpower to stage the huge function at the Pixler mansion, the *Larkspur Ledger* screamed with ads soliciting temporary help. The promotions flaunted the contributing businesses and the available secondary work opportunities as if someone might as well work free simply to be associated with the once-in-a-lifetime, charitable extravaganza. All that hype was in preparation for the usual minimum wage that would be doled out to the temp employees, one of which was sure to be Wayne Simmons.

"Couldn't care less what they're gonna pay," Wayne said as he popped the newspaper with his right index finger, knowing that he would easily get a job with one of the catering companies. The salary was not important to Wayne Simmons. All he needed was a means to get into that house, that large house that according to his client needed torching really badly. He was not sure why his client wanted it torched, but then he never asked why. That was none of his business.

Wayne carried a portfolio of fake resumes qualifying him for varied positions, having downloaded them from unsecured internet websites. He updated his collection with computer research at the Larkspur Library, finding a curriculum vitae for food service work that was especially thorough, laid out especially neatly. The fools at the principal catering firm would accept his application; he was sure of it. No matter how bogus, the references would go unquestioned as would his impeccable interview appearance to parallel the impressive resume. Before the catering job interview he would mousse his hair, leave a little fashionable facial stubble, wear some tight pants, fake an English accent, and be prepared for whoever or whatever was accepting the applications.

The confusion associated with organizing such a grand event was inevitable, as inevitable as its ostentatious nature which would rise to equal the ostentatious site of the party. Wayne understood all that, and many times before he had played that disorder to his advantage. That disorder would be the preliminary diversion needed for his setup. Once Simmons was part of the catering team, slipping the candles in with the food and beverage supply deliveries would be effortless and go unnoticed by those in charge. Those bosses would be engrossed in perfecting fresh flower arrangements, positioning ice sculptures just so, and stringing delicate white lights all over the place – in the bushes, entwined in the intricate ironwork of the façade and lining the walkways throughout the gardens of the property – a decoration that Wayne believed should be reserved for Christmastime. "That's too damn sacrilegious," he would say to himself that night.

During his trial drive-by, Wayne had wondered why anyone would want a home that outsized and detailed. "Too much damn trouble to keep up a place like that." However, its design as a matter of taste was not a concern to him. The large estate appeared newly constructed and with its freshly installed foundation plantings seemed to represent a lot of upkeep to him. His commentary on the Pixler mansion was made out of pure curiosity as he sized up the place, more out of professional observation than criticism.

The monstrous house would be overflowing with gawking hungry and thirsty guests as ostentatious as their surroundings, Wayne thought. The arsonist's assumption was that the hosts would plan to satiate the throng by scattering multiple food and beverage stations throughout, and those stations would require volumes of supplies and many deliveries. Those many deliveries would be the answer.

The client had agreed to a pricey commission upon being promised a thorough job, a flawless one. *I want the whole place gone, burned to a crisp* were the exact words. The client networking that had landed him this Larkspur project had been built upon his reputation for perfectionism, a status he meant to uphold. To accomplish the order calling for complete destruction by fire in the guise of accident, he would count on the Party Happy candle in every shape and color.

First, he would need to get the little beauties onsite and in position. "Easy, easy. This will be a piece of cake," he told himself as he stopped for a moment to make a few notes, using the pen and paper pad he had also just purchased at the discount store. Once the caterer's spread of food and liquor was laid out at the party, he would slip the pretty candles among the organized decorative clutter. No one would see him for all the scurrying about: workers bumping into other workers carrying heavy trays of expensive, smelly fodder meant to be more gorgeous than edible, all the while cursing mostly under their collective breaths instead of paying proper attention to what a lowly extra like Wayne Simmons was doing. For once, Wayne's cockiness over the ingenuity of his own blueprint surprised even him, particularly since most of his jobs were accomplished in the dark without anyone around.

Squelching any last minute misgivings and reaching into his pocket to finger the job's payment, he said defiantly, "Nobody will stop me from what I'm doing during setup; in fact, I'm sure nobody'll even notice. Hell, it'll be a damn goat circus around that house."

Chapter

23

•••

THE SQUIRRELS

Again I followed the advice Kaylee had given me that day in the food market and repeatedly attempted to call my grandfather to check on him. He had never carried a cellphone on his person but did keep one in the car, never bothering to activate the voice mail to any of his phones. When my landline as well as cellular calls continued to go unanswered, I assumed he was not staying at home much or doing much driving around. Besides, where did he have to go? According to Mr. Desselle, he wasn't even hitting the links anymore.

He had employed a new housekeeper of sorts a few years ago, certainly not one as wonderful as the late Chrissie Funchess. Nevertheless, I assumed the current maid would have sense enough to notify the next of kin or at least call the police upon discovering her employer dead or missing. Therefore, I expected no morbid surprise as I drove to the house in Manorwood Heights. Because my grandfather's state of depression had destroyed any semblance of happiness for me there, I really did not want to return to that aging spread and to what was left of my childhood home.

Selfishly, I tossed aside any of Granddad's concern over what I had done with my life. That's what it was after all: my life. And I was the child; I would be the one who would live it. Once coming to that understanding, I believed that our next face-to-face encounter would be less painful, at least for me. How he would be affected was anyone's guess.

As I kept the Mustang pointed up my grandfather's driveway that evening, I wondered whether I would find him in the den or the study. He might be sitting in a dusty leather chair and watching his home video collage in the dark or perhaps crying over the photo albums by the light of a dim lamp. That possibility was what I dreaded most – witnessing my only relative continuing to relive the former happiness of his family's innocent, ignorant days.

Why hadn't Senior just answered the phone when I called repeatedly? Then I would have been off the hook with Kaylee and my own conscience – Kaylee, for sure, my conscience, maybe. Nevertheless, she was right. Kaylee was always right. I needed to see my lonely grandfather, and I believed he would want to see me.

Kaylee's disgust at her boyfriend's avoidance of his own grandfather was pushing me up to the top of the driveway. A reversed course that day would have certainly earned the horrified rebuke of her slow and painful punishment. My spine stiffened as I successfully fought the urge to return to my apartment for a drink or two, maybe three. I simply dreaded seeing my grandfather's sad, dehydrated eyes, eyes drained of tears shed for all of his losses. Though not exactly on course, my life was by contrast still ahead – all the unknowns that had manifested themselves as brutal, morbid events in my grandfather's life were still positive chances for me. I knew of no other person in Larkspur, or anywhere else for that matter, who had survived an only son and daughter-in-law while witnessing the slow, deteriorating demise of his own wife.

At that point in my life, regardless of Kaylee's good intentions for my actions, I knew there was nothing I could say to Granddad that could ease his mental suffering and regret. Was there anything that could give solace to an old man like that, I remember wondering. My getting into medical school – would that do it? Is that what I could tell the med school admissions committee during an interview: please let me be a physician so that I can make my miserable grandfather happy?

There was no response to the doorbell and a firm rapping of the heavy, brass knocker that followed likewise went unanswered. With each impatient knock, my horror mounted that the worthless housekeeper had skipped work for a few days, leaving my deceased grandfather to develop rigor mortis in that dusty leather chair, family photos having fallen askew from his arms to the floor. That image pierced my chest to the hilt, that of a grandson too cowardly to confront a grieving, depressing grandfather.

When my repeated pounding of the front door went unanswered, I realized that it was well past the maid's quitting time and that only my grandfather should be there to answer. His car was not parked in the front bay. He never left it there, always pulling it into the garage, a habit attributed as much to appearances as safety. I walked around to the side of the house where the attached, windowless multi-car garage stood, finding all of the doors tightly shut and impossible to raise from the exterior without the electric opener.

My right hand found its way nervously into my pants pocket, searching for the main house key that I knew was there, the one left over from high school when my bankrupt family moved into the poolhouse section of the complex. Until then there had been a foreboding sense of dread preventing me from again using the key, except I knew that I should check on my grandfather.

Opening his front door released not a rush of air but instead a clear, enveloping odor that was not as stale as expected. By definition, the aura of an old person's house is certain to have a degree of stagnation, not necessarily an offensive smell, unless, of course, the home overflows with the infirmed and all associated with it.

"Granddad!" I called, actually yelled, after I cleared my throat when at first I could not speak. There was no answer because there was no way he could have heard me.

The grand entrance foyer of the Foxworth home pushes through to the back of the house where it ends perpendicular to an expansive windowed room used as a den. It was down that wide corridor and through those opened windows that I could see my grandfather. He was standing in the back gardens, far enough from the main house to be out of earshot of the door bell and my yelling.

Walking to the back of the house toward him, I passed the recessed bookcases that mark the den entrance. As expected, the shelving was lined with photographs of Foxworths and their friends, and unlike those in my father's old room, these frames were dusted and supported shining glass covers. One picture stood askew from the others, its protective glass uniquely marred by fingerprints. It was of the three of us: Mom, me, and Dad. We had been to the Larkspur Mall on a Saturday afternoon; I guess I was in the sixth or seventh grade then. Dad had suggested that we stop to get a vendor to photograph us, saying something about my grandparents wanting a more recent picture. The small, informal family portrait would become a favorite of my grandfather. I had not seen that photograph in years, so I picked up the oval wood and glass frame, mixing my fingerprints with those undoubtedly belonging to Granddad.

All three of us were smiling – my mom looking down at me, my dad and I toward the camera. We were all happy and so unsuspecting.

Realigning the framed photograph back on the shelf with the others, I next moved through the den to exit the rear French doors. The old man turned reflexively, not at all startled, as I called out in greeting, "Hey, Granddad. Howya been?"

"Sher, my boy! A visit?" His tone was more of surprise than question. "How are things at the fire department?"

"Pretty quiet lately. In fact, I've had some time off to do some other things."

"Oh, yes. Girlfriend things."

"No, well, yes. That, too. You see, I shawdowed this doctor over in Montclair that Kaylee knows. Actually, he's her doctor, tried to get a little feel of what practicing medicine would be like. I think Kaylee hoped the exposure would get my interest revved up for trying to get into medical school again."

"And did it?"

My affirmative answer came a little too quickly for even me to believe its sincerity. Truthfully, I was still uncertain that I wanted to pursue the route of being any kind of physician, certainly not that of a gynecologist like Knox Chamblee.

"You know, Sher," continued my closest blood relative, "your decision needs to be based not on what I want for you or even what your girl wants for you or, perhaps, wants for herself, but instead should be made after you sort through your fears."

"Fears?"

At some time during the exchange Granddad had turned away from me and was gazing out into the backyard. There were no photo albums or home movies anywhere around. Thick with low-limbed oak trees draped with Spanish moss and other shrubbery, the area was coated in various green hues but was void of other colors that would have served to break the monotony of the landscape. It was as though the planted space professed that life must be sustained even without anything blooming, even without any brightness.

The stillness of the deep backyard was broken only by the antics of the neighborhood squirrels, many of which seemed to have based themselves on the Foxworth property.

"Yes, fears," Granddad replied. "If you decide not to resume the application process for medical school, I'm concerned it will be out of fear of another rejection, I hope, more so that your being concerned about all the hard work required to get there and stay there. Of course, that doesn't include the working lifestyle required after finishing medical training. That in itself can be cause enough to back away. I remember how your father once shared with me his sense of feeling overwhelmed after he was finally out of medical school and finished with all that other training. He had successfully completed all the legal work to establish his surgical group (and there was lots of paperwork, I recall) and was facing the challenge of building a booming practice in plastics ... " His voice trailed off sadly as the squirrels scampered unabashed from limb to limb, and I worked to ease the awkwardness of our own exchange.

I struggled to continue the unique openness of that conversation between us. My efforts may have seemed forced, but I tried my best. There was no opportunity for me to have a conversation of this nature with anyone else since my parents had been taken from me at a time when most teenagers would have, given the choice, figuratively erased their parents. Positioned before me looking out into nature was my only living parent of any type, and in the absence of my dead mother and father, I had shamefully let dissipate the opportunity for him to assume a greater role in my life.

As he remained silent, I replayed his last words in my mind. Maybe he was correct. Maybe I was too afraid, too fearful, of what medical school acceptance would require of me. Maybe that's why I blew my freshman year academically at Ole Miss, but maybe I was just too immature then.

Had fighting fires and saving lives in that manner built character for me since? Probably not, since the blazes around Larkspur had lacked that kind of drama. Time had built any character I possessed, as the true impact of my family losses had grown into my psyche, hardening it somewhat.

This elderly but still handsome man, who had physically held up well during the years even if not emotionally, loved me deeply and wanted me to make more of myself. I knew that. I knew that all along and was growing to believe that his wishes were not really for himself or for my dead parents, but instead for me.

I worked at a believable response and was successful from my perspective. "Granddad, I guess I've always seen myself as a doctor but lacked the maturity to get there. But I believe I know now, actually I'm sure that I know now what I've got to do. It won't be easy, but ... " Those were words that would have satisfied most elders of wayward progeny; however, my grandfather said nothing, as my voice was the one that trailed this time. In contrast, he seemed to nod his head slightly in agreement and acceptance, looking back toward me before returning to study the terrain of his backyard.

My pause was a fraction too long, and Granddad spoke instead. "We have suffered so much around here, Sher, and who's to blame for it? Most of the time when I get like this I want to blame that Pixler fella for all of the family's misfortune. His driving your parents into the ground financially is not what killed them, I know. But I never thought your Dad was the same after the malpractice verdict and the failed appeals. He seemed so distracted, so lost. Losing his plastic surgery practice and seeing his partners leave town was equal to losing the one thing he had worked for his whole life. It wasn't just the money; it was his pride. I should never have let him start flying again. Hell, he was a grown man. You can't tell a grown man what to do, even if he is your son." I looked down at my feet, knowing I was a prime example of that school of thought.

"I'm sorry, Son. I certainly don't need to point out the family's misfortune to you. After all, you were the poor boy who lost his parents. But I have held it all inside myself, moping all day long even in front of you when you'd come over to visit me. Which really hasn't been all that often," he added with a sly smile. "All you've seen me do is cry over the loss of my only child – really the loss of my only children, since I loved Kathleen as a daughter. I've barely swung a golf club in the last few months except for one afternoon over in Montclair."

"Now, that's really a bad sign. What's the world comin' to?" I responded in a feeble attempt at comic relief, an effort which went unnoticed.

"When I'm not sitting inside, I sometimes stand or sit on this patio for hours like it's a prison, watching these damn squirrels living out their lives, fancy-free. I've become envious of them: chasing each other, probably trying to mate, not a care in the world except where the next acorn is coming from. There are so many of the damn flea-bitten things, running all over the place, all over the patio furniture and those brick walls over there." He pointed to the short pediments which defined the stonework of the patio. "Sometimes I feel like the squirrels are watching me, trying to return the favor as though my life is as interesting as theirs." Although at that moment I could not see his eyes, I felt them, the tone of his voice seeming to reflect a parallel sign of resolution. "Sher, I know what I want to do now – I know what I have to do now."

I said nothing since I didn't know what to say. I wished for Kaylee and her knack for kindness. She would have known what to say to this sad, broken man. I think I remember a tear or two falling to my cheek as I wished that I had not gone over to

Granddad's house that day, but instead had remained cowardly and let more and more weeks go by.

A large squirrel, not really fatter than the others, just more robust and obviously well-coordinated, suddenly leaped from the oak limb closest to the patio and scampered along the entire length of the squatty brick wall, his tail thick and slightly stubby as though muscular like the rest of his torso. "That's Rocky; he sort of reminds me of Sylvester Stallone." Granddad glanced over to me as he introduced us. "And that's Lauren. She's a dead ringer for Lauren Bacall." He motioned to a svelte, almost blonde-colored squirrel that had joined Rocky in the ring, trying to claim the berries clinging to a holly bush that grew at the foot of the bricked enclosure. The second squirrel reminded me more of Gwyneth Paltrow but my last attempt at comic relief had died, so I dropped it.

Instead, I became speechless, praying Granddad would not introduce me to any more of the furry creatures that had become his life. Like my grandfather, I knew then that I had to do something, something for him, something for me.

Turning to leave, I said goodbye to a truly emotionally and apparently mentally destroyed man and wished that I had not returned to a place that was no longer a home.

Chapter
24

•••

THE CALL

We parked in the lot of a neighboring upscale shopping center and rode the shuttle to the fundraiser for the Larkspur Institute for Education. Because of the limited parking area in Manorwood Heights, various automobile dealerships in and around Larkspur and Montclair had donated new cars and drivers to transport the paying guests to the Pixler home. Although the cause was charitable, the homeowners in that exclusive neighborhood would rightly frown upon tire tracks marring their pristine lawns, regardless if the tires supported a Mercedes, BMW, Lexus, Cadillac, as well as Bentley or Rolls. Kaylee and I were not paying guests but were riding the coattails of her father, who had given us his ticket for two, and we were fortunate enough to snatch a ride in a Hummer stretch limo, a first for us both.

The relatively short ride to the Pixler Palace took us through the narrow, curvy streets of Manorwood Estates, an obstacle course at times for a standard-sized vehicle, much less our limo. To our surprise, as well as that of the other partygoers spaced inside the Hummer, the driver delicately navigated the immense vehicle around the blooming azaleas, erupting ferns, clustered pansies,

and budding dogwoods which closely lined the asphalt streets.
Soon the city flower larkspur would grace the flower beds of the
Manorwood Heights and elsewhere.

Kaylee and I noticed few homeowners in their front yards.
Few would be expected to be out doing yard work anyway, but
generally some residents would be walking or jogging around the
neighborhood at this time of evening. However, the desolation of
any neighborhood activity except for that associated with the party
itself was really no surprise. Anybody who was anyone or wanted
to be someone wouldn't be stuck at home in their own manor that
night. Instead, they would be joining us at the social occasion of
the year, maybe of the decade.

As we rounded the final corner to the estate, I envisioned the
smoke and ash rising from Mrs. Architzel's old house that once
stood in place of the Pixler's pride-and-joy, a showplace awaiting
its introduction into southern society. While my eyes focused on
the replacement structure rising from the peak of that hill, its
massive front door crowning a path of steps from the street, I
could almost hear Dickens' alarming, chirping bark.

"Sher, we're here," Kaylee whispered as she nudged me toward
the door of the limo and back to the present. Having been the last
couple to be seated in the vehicle, we were closest to its main exit,
and in my daydreaming I had not noticed the tuxedoed driver
waiting to help us out. As I escorted Kaylee from the Hummer, the
memory of Dickens's shrill yap was replaced by the sound of dance
band music, so loud that a street party for the entire neighborhood
could have been possible. "Come on, Hunk. Let's get inside, have a
drink, and dance," Kaylee said as she walked me to the front steps
of the Pixler Palace.

As instructed when hired by the caterer, Wayne rode in his
designated van to the job, arriving about an hour before the bash
was to start. He felt debonair in the starched white monogrammed

uniform on loan from the owner of the company with the understanding that the outfit had to be left with her after the party cleanup was completed. "No returned uniform, no pay," she had warned. When she added, "We can also charge you with stealing if you don't make the return," Wayne wondered what kind of low-life help the owner usually hired. To draw as little attention to himself as possible, Simmons planned to follow the instructions exactly, just as he had done up to that moment. Of course, when the time came for the pre-party bedlam accompanying the last minute touches, he would forget the boss lady's demands and put his alternative plans in place.

A back corner of the Pixler property abutted a short, hidden street that was actually an access alley for the next door neighbor's rear drive. Unlike the hustle and bustle of the Pixler acreage, Wayne had discovered while casing the site that the house and grounds next door were empty, deserted. Wayne noted that the expansive yard still showed signs of a once beautiful landscape but that the huge rose garden stood as unkempt and overgrown as the rest of the place. He wondered how long the large house had been abandoned and how long it would be before someone called him to take care of it.

One section of the garage belonging to the adjacent unoccupied house, the part closest to the Pixler property line, was enclosed by a door that could be manually raised from the outside, a finding that Wayne found careless from a security standpoint even if the space was empty. The day before the party he filled his rental car with gas and stored it there in preparation for his escape once the house was ablaze. Initially he planned to stash his Wal-Mart supplies behind his car, just inside the closed garage door. At the last minute he changed plans, hiding them in a spacious covered cabinet located around the corner from the garage that contained only a few rusted, abandoned garden tools.

The Party Happy candles and other ignition source paraphernalia, which included brake fluid for the coffee maker canisters, would lie in wait for him until the next day. The secure storage site was close enough in proximity that he should be able to slip away unmissed from his service assignment to retrieve his arson supplies. Wayne had found only one hitch in this scheme: an obstacle in the form of a tall, ancient cyclone fence that enclosed that particular rear corner of the Pixler estate, barely visible under an encasement of tangled dark green ivy. During his snooping around before the big day, Wayne had judged the barrier to be a manageable climb, especially for someone as compact and agile as he and particularly with no dogs around to chase him.

Faith Behneman was pleased that the manager of the catering firm had assigned her to the lead van of their service entourage since she would be afforded more time in the house. Impressing the manager and getting the job as a catering assistant had been simple, using her new resume, which detailed experience assisting in the production of beauty pageants and the like. The document, fluffed up quite a bit with references that would never be verified, looked polished after she drafted it with the aid of a computer at the Larkspur Library. A young, pretty librarian there, oblivious to Faith's true intentions, had been extremely helpful to her in completing and printing the document.

To use for the job, she had purchased an oversized purse at Wal-Mart that resembled a demure-appearing beach bag more so than a ladie's handbag. She then added a small overnight carryall to her personal things. "Looks like you're loaded down there," observed the nosy man with the slight build as he entered the van, choosing the seat next to Faith. Like Faith, he was wearing the same style white caterer's uniform on loan from the manager.

At first Faith decided to ignore him but then realized it might be less conspicuous to answer. "Yvette told me we were to turn in the uniform tonight when we're through with the party and cleanup, so I brought a change of clothes."

This explanation did not satisfy Wayne Simmons as he continued to stare curiously at the two bags, while Faith grew more self-conscious. Beginning to become nervous, she wondered why he was shaking his head at her bags as though he was almost coveting them. Unknown to Faith, Wayne had begun to shake his head in disgust over the lost opportunity. Already fearful that he was faced with more than two trips from his clandestine storage site on the other side of that ivy-covered fence, he realized he could have utilized the same type of gear to transport not clothes, but arson supplies instead.

Feeling guilty and made more so as the meddlesome man shook his head, Faith expounded, "Oh, uhh, I'm carrying a lot of stuff – makeup, nice clothes, and stuff like that. Uhh, I'm going to another function after we get off – another party, to party for myself, that is." Afraid that she was digging herself into a situation that could lead to another unwanted problem, she clarified, "I'm meeting my husband at the party. We're both really looking forward to it." As she stammered and stumbled, Faith noticed that the man had spied her ringless wedding ring finger. She corrected clumsily, "I mean, I'm meeting my boyfriend." Whatever the talkative woman's social problems or plans, Wayne was not interested in them or her. He continued silently to berate himself for not toting a portion of his professional stuff in such bags.

The man seemed content with her explanation and thankfully stopped asking questions or conversing in any other manner. Faith then turned her own attention to the precious cargo resting between her legs and also between her and the intrusive man. Fortunately for Faith, the head caterer's large white van had decent shocks, and due to a recent repaving, the roads through that section of Manorwood Heights were smooth. As a result, her treasure went undisturbed throughout the ride. Faith Behneman's two heavy cloth carriers stored as many clear plastic airtight containers as she could stuff into them. Another product of Wal-Mart, the containers were commonly available heavy plastic boxes and jars equipped with easily removable but firmly secured, airtight lids. Faith had chosen the products because of their light weight when empty. After all, when filled with gasoline they were heavy enough.

"Mind if I smoke?" Simmons asked loudly enough for every van passenger to hear. A smoke before a job served to calm his nerves and collect his thoughts. "I can roll down this window here and you'll never know it."

"For God's sake, no!" Faith almost screamed her response but quickly retreated into modest indignation. The other temps riding in the front section of the van were in agreement but still were taken back by the harsh tone of her voice. Just as Wayne Simmons, they were ignorant to the possibility of being engulfed in a rolling inferno should Faith's plastic containers fail as airtight.

Wayne stared at her with eyes that spoke words not used in mixed company, and she sensed developing anger. Faith stumbled again, "I mean we're almost there ... to the party, that is. See there's the house up the street, and we can't arrive smelling of cigarette smoke. Yvette will fire us on the spot. And, frankly, I don't know about you," she continued while clutching her treasure and looking around the van pleading for support in her debate, "I need the work – got bills to pay."

Further debate was unnecessary as the van pulled up the hill to the rear parking area of the Pixler house. The driver followed the manager's directive in parking the van clearly out of sight. No one wanted to cross Yvette.

As soon as everyone disembarked and scattered to their assigned posts, Wayne disappeared unnoticed through the shrubbery to the back of the property. As he moved to retrieve his supplies, Faith Behneman carefully unloaded her own ignition source and headed toward the house with her bags.

"Miss, I overhead what you were saying about going somewhere later," the van driver, a fulltime employee of Yvette's Catering Service, called out to Faith. As he continued she was so startled that she nearly dropped the heaviest of her hazardous load. "You can leave your change of clothes in here and get them after the party cleanup. The van will be locked up real tight until we're finished and can leave."

"Damn," Faith said under her breath. "Can't anyone mind their own stinkin' business?"

"Your stuff'll be safe here 'til you need it, I promise. Those bags look heavy. Why do you want to carry them around anyway?"

Out of fear that the busybody driver might suddenly become chivalrous, jumping to help her with the bags and discovering their contents, Faith nervously fought to balance them between both arms. That was not a simple task combined with trying to steady herself after stepping from the van. "Oh, I'll be fine," she responded almost before he completed the offer. "This stuff really won't take up that much room inside, and I'll be able to find a place for it. In fact, I know just where to put it 'cause I've worked this place before," she lied as she scurried with great care through the nearby back entrance of the Pixler Palace.

The lie was in her claim that she had worked at the Pixler residence, but in truth she had been there previously, if only in the virtual sense. The broadcast television home tours which had run repeatedly as part of the aggressive media campaign had enabled Faith to plan exactly where she was to store the gasoline at the fundraiser, except she would not store it in the inexpensive plastic containers. The expensive, soft European comforters covering the upstairs and master bedroom beds would store the gasoline nicely as they readily soaked it up — so would the thick, multi-layered living and dining room draperies that the television news anchorwoman had fawned over in disguised envy.

Once everyone was busy displaying the food and putting the final touches on the flower arrangements and other decorations, Faith planned to move through the house unnoticed, tossing gasoline in a vengeful spree, starting in any unoccupied upstairs bedroom and moving quickly, stealthily downstairs to the other planned targets. The side pockets of her white caterer's uniform were filled with small, plastic cigarette lighters that she would toss at the gasoline-marred fabrics.

Faith was smiling, almost laughing, in delightful anticipation. Finally she would realize retribution for her ruined family. The doctor had been long punished, and now Lawyer Pixler's fine, blood-money house would meet the same satisfying end. Even if the house was not annihilated by her actions that night, she was convinced the damage would be extensive, heartbreaking for Pixler and his no-doubt trashy bimbo of a wife.

"Good, you're finally here." Yvette nearly yanked Faith's left arm out of socket as she pulled the temp from the laundry room where Faith had stashed gasoline laden bags. "Girl, I need you to come in here right now," Yvette continued with direction, "and get this dining room table straightened out."

"But, I, ah, I need to ... "

"You **need** to follow me into the dining room. According to that resume you gave the agency, your specialty is food arrangement. So, after you get everything spruced up in there, I want you to stand at the head of the table to serve the bisque and make sure it stays replenished. That crab meat concoction is my dear husband's specialty. It's always popular, a real crowd-pleaser, and will go real fast. Besides we need someone sort of attractive in that spot and you, Sweetie, are unfortunately the best I've got here in that regard."

"But, ah, I was going to ... " Yvette continued to ignore the pleas as the two made it to the banquet-sized dining room.

"I'll have one of the others working in the kitchen keep the sterling basin filled for you. All you'll have to do is smile pretty, be polite, keep stirring the wonderful crab bisque, and make sure the warmer under the basin stays lit," Yvette summarized emphatically as she used her own lighter to ignite the can of heating fluid positioned directly under the bowl.

The erupting flame was much, much smaller than Faith had planned.

"Good evening, Mr. and Mrs. King," the doorman greeted us, reading Kaylee's family name from her father's original invitation. Fire Marshal Lisenbe's moniker stood distinctly with the other engraving that seemed to spring from the thick off-white parchment bordered in Larkspur Institute for Education colors.

"Oh, we're not ... " I was interrupted by a nudge from Kaylee's elbow, since the salutation really did not matter. We were there with her father's gift of a paid invitation that would have otherwise become landfill, and she was going to have a blast with her handsome boyfriend.

"Can you believe this place," we exclaimed almost in unison, our remarks falling on ears nearly deafened by the roar of feasting, drinking, gossiping and dancing partygoers. Even though the band was playing in the back, the music flowed unabated through the tall, fully opened French doors that lined the rear of the mansion. I glanced across the crowd to check out the performance coming from a slightly raised sundeck at the pool's center. Giving the illusion of floating in the middle of the tranquil water, Pinkie and the Panthers were the bomb for the delirious crowd. Modern in musical style although outfitted in formal evening wear, the musicians were belting out hits from several decades as a gyrating storm of revelers surrounded them on the patio.

To the right of the custom-designed pool were Mrs. Architzel's sweet olive bushes, still thriving and fortunate to have been growing in a spot that escaped the property's earlier fate. Their leaves remained deeply green and so thick that the mature plants merely blended into the darkness, the sweet-olive aroma lost to the air intoxicated for dissimilar reasons. Nearby, G.G. Gerbing azaleas provided a blanketing contrast. Spring blossoms had come early, and the heavy, bright white flowers appeared iridescent as though lit with fluorescent lighting hanging camouflaged in the trees above. With distinction, delicate white dogwood petals filled a rear corner, like individual snowflakes scattered among the layers of established trees and shrubbery.

"Sher, I know you're hungry, but I'd really like to dance." Kaylee touched me suggestively as she again returned me to the present, her intimacy unnoticed by everyone else as they were deep into their own self-satisfaction.

"I'd like to do whatever you want to do," I responded with just as much intimacy, "but I'll have a lot more energy to do whatever that turns out to be if we grab a little grub first."

"Then you have my permission to eat," she acquiesced, "but do it fast."

We made our way through the crowd to an immense, oblong mahogany table that was the final resting place for many, many trees. Manning the top of the table and opposite us was a somewhat unhappy-looking woman, dressed in a caterer's uniform that nearly matched her colorless skin. She was serving a soup of some kind to a growing line of hungry-looking men who resembled the Depression-era unemployed, except that they were tuxedo-clad and held gold-rimmed china bowls with sterling silver spoons.

Throughout the food table display, each edible was labeled by name so that there was no way to miss either its delicacy or the name of its creator. First we approached the fried calamari that guarded a dipping sauce described as zesty that was followed by another appetizer in the form of martini glasses overflowing with fresh ceviche marinated in lime juice and herbs. Since I had not yet been to the bar to get us a drink and no server had made his way toward us, we decided that we were not ready for zesty or raw fish, no matter whose secret family recipe claimed it. However, the caramelized brie with spiced pecans and the goat cheese and sun-dried tomato crostini which followed looked more inviting to me.

"Oh, look, these are oysters in pastry shells. The card says that they're creamy," Kaylee announced as she picked the largest one and pushed it between my lips. The sauce lacing the plump oyster was indeed creamy, made all the more rich by Kaylee's forefinger pushing it against my tongue. As I chewed and swallowed, she, as expected, skipped that heavy seafood delicacy. Girls really don't eat at parties, anyway.

As if at a swanky cafeteria, we made slow progress down the feeding line to the center of our side of the table. An obese man in a chef's hat was diligently frying what looked like oversized egg rolls. My first thought regarding the sight was that I would never have allowed anyone to fry anything on my own mahogany table, much less allow it to be done in a formal room complete with priceless wallpaper and rugs. Nevertheless, the fellow appeared to know what he was doing, handling the pan and utensil with precise surgical skill while producing no noticeable plume or spattered grease.

"What are these?" I inquired of the chef, not waiting to receive a response before presenting my plate for a fill.

"Mississippi Rolls, my wife Yvette's specialty. That's her over there." He gestured with a metal spatula toward an authoritative woman who had stopped by the crab bisque to check on the server's status. There seemed to be a minor argument between the two, but Yvette left apparently victorious, the server looking more disgruntled.

"Mississippi Roll?" coming up immediately behind us, Kaylee was showing interest.

"Yes, these are exquisitely thin crispy Mississippi Delta catfish filets driven in from Belzoni. We got them fresh out of the pond, and then rolled the prepared fillets in sushi, mixing in the perfect amount of avocado and spicy aioli. The exact amount of each ingredient is a secret that Yvette has shared only with me, of course." As the rotund chef gingerly placed a Mississippi Roll on my china plate, he added with a wink at Kaylee, "The spicy aioli recipe is under wraps as well."

Both of us enthusiastically took a bite of our portion of the treasured delicacy, smiling happily while chewing in an exaggerated show of great gratitude to the fellow for sharing the treat with us. "Sher, this really is good," Kaylee said. "Might even be an aphrodisiac," she winked.

"Let's hope so. Maybe you should go back for seconds."

"That won't be necessary," she clarified with lips coated in a thin layer of the spicy aioli that she sensuously licked clean with her tongue.

After clearing my throat at the thought, I suggested, "Let's find the bar."

Kaylee followed in agreement as we pulled out of the hungry line, leaving behind the fresh lump crabmeat and capers drizzled with Meyer truffle oil on crispy toast points. Neither would we gorge on the beef tenderloin, the fresh Atlantic smoked salmon, nor the succulent lamb chops crusted with fresh rosemary and ground black and red pepper accompanied with homemade mint jelly.

We worked our way into the next room, past the swarm with full plates trying to balance a cocktail glass, linen napkin, and a silver fork while buzzing tall tales. Still we spotted no bar in this space which appeared to be a breakfast or morning room of sorts, offering an instant case of diabetes mellitus. As in the dining room, each offering was labeled. Continuation of this pattern by the party's organizers was fortunate because I for one would not have recognized most of the dessert concoctions. Such items as individual caramel doberge cakes, truffles sprinkled with edible gold dust, chocolate whiskey cake with fresh mint chocolate sauce and whiskey ice cream, bananas foster fried pie with homemade rum ice cream, and individual servings of tiramisu covered every available surface in the room. There was not a cobbler or a scoop of plain vanilla ice cream to be found, and I looked.

As thirsty Kaylee and I continued to explore, we finally found that one of the rear French doors led directly to the outside where a small bar awaited. Off the main drag of revelers, it was not as busy as the other areas; it simply had not been noticed yet. As I got in line for our cocktails, Kaylee waited off to the side where she began to move her feet and swing her shoulders gently to the band music.

"Granddad!" The tall, tuxedoed gentleman ahead of me in line turned around holding two gin-and-tonic cocktails. "Granddad!" I repeated with even more surprise, realizing I was not hallucinating from an overdose of dietary sugar and fatty food.

"Sher, I didn't know you would be here!" he interjected with equal astonishment.

"Gosh, I would never have expected you to get anywhere close to Cordell ... "

"Let me introduce you to my date, My Boy," he interrupted as though he had heard nothing I had just said. I forced my mouth closed and forgot the cocktails as I followed him over to an attractive, well-preserved woman (no, I should say *lady*) standing coincidentally near Kaylee. She looked thirty years younger than Senior, but I suspected that it was only a twenty-year difference. "Madelyn, I would like for you to meet my grandson, Sheridan Foxworth III. But we've always called him Sher." In regal fashion the lady extended an impeccably manicured left hand, sporting a diamond that even my mother would have thought too large. However, I doubt if Kathleen Foxworth would have refused the opportunity to wear it.

"Sher, this is Madelyn Gwinn, my fiancée."

Had I been holding a cocktail glass, it would have been in pieces on the patio. Wisely, I had asked Kaylee to hold my dinner plate when I got in the short bar line, or pieces of fine white china mixed with remnants of a Mississippi Roll would have decorated the stone surface. By then, Kaylee had noticed my talking with Granddad and recognized him although they had only met once before.

"Mr. Foxworth. Hi! Kaylee Lisenbe. It's wonderful to see you again." As she explained to me later, my girlfriend noticed the facial pallor and little beads of sweat around my mouth and on my forehead despite the dim lighting draping across the patio and pool area of the Pixler Palace.

"Hello, Miss Lisenbe. I'm delighted to see you again as well. Please let me introduce you to Madelyn Gwinn." Kaylee turned and extended her hand with a gorgeous smile. "You may know her as *Mrs. Cullen Gwinn*. Madelyn is from Montclair. Her late husband was a physician over there, a gynecologist."

"Yes, my dear Cullen passed away a while back," Mrs. Gwinn clarified. "I met Sheridan one afternoon when he was over at the Montclair Club playing golf. He and I happened to be having massages the same afternoon."

"Madelyn, you might want to clarify that a bit. We weren't

having a couple's massage, at least not then." They both laughed and the couple I would never have expected nudged closer to each other as Kaylee and I subconsciously stepped back.

"Sher," Granddad turned toward me with a slightly more sober attitude but with nevertheless the grin of someone in a happy place. "Over the past several weeks, Madelyn and I have been seeing a lot of each other. We were both lonely but somehow were drawn to each other."

"Your grandfather is a wonderful man, and, Sher, I see that you have inherited his good looks," Mrs. Gwinn, the woman I would learn to call Madelyn, purred with a comforting smile that immediately explained my grandfather's earlier decision: *Sher, I know what I want to do now – I know what I have to do now.*

That day on his patio, surrounded by squirrels and deep in solemn thought, he had decided not to forget my grandmother or my parents, but to move on with his life.

"Don't you two want to join us youngsters on the dance floor? Madelyn bought these tickets and tempted me to come with her for the dancing. There are so many people here, you can just avoid the undesirables – particularly the attorneys, if you know what I mean!" Granddad almost joked as he whisked Mrs. Gwinn away to the sounds of Pinkie and the Panthers. The ensemble sounded surprisingly together, their music resonating from the sundeck in the center of the pool, enlivening the entire shoulder-to-shoulder crowd heating up the rear patio. Thirsting for emotional relief from that heart-stopping surprise, I hurriedly ran back to the bar to grab a scotch and water for myself and a glass of chardonnay for Kaylee. As we followed the "youngsters" toward the main throng of dancers, my drink was downed in no more than two gulps, and I needed a refill badly.

In the center of the crowd were a man and woman, again he older than she, but clearly a generation or so younger than the

Foxworth–Gwinn match. As he spun her around and unknowingly faced me, I recognized him: Pixler, the devil himself. No, he was more than the devil. He was an asshole. His life was more than good by earthly standards: elaborate home, sexy wife, lots of money, no immediate family rotting in graves anywhere, at least none that I knew of.

Pixler never recognized me, or my grandfather. He was too drunk, or too high or whatever, to be aware of much more than the firm, young bosoms shaking before him, barely supported by a dress made more of jewels than fabric. Boy, was that pair having a blast.

Cordell and Rachel Pixler were oblivious to everyone around them although they were in their beloved element. Their subjects surrounded them in revelry; they had made it.

No one appreciated them more than Gregory Whitestone and the president of the foundation. I did not spot Eugene McNabb in the masses, but missing Whitestone was impossible. He was dancing near the Pixlers, probably to keep a lurid eye on the youthful missus. The monetary success of the night's fundraiser would no doubt lead to a higher headmaster's salary although the gyration before him in the form of nimble Rachel Pixler was at the moment payment enough.

As Kaylee and I danced alongside my grandfather and his date, we, like the blissfully intoxicated Pixlers and Gregory Whitestone, failed to notice the striking woman who had pushed her way through the burgeoning multitude to stare at Cordell and Rachel. She was drinking not from the glassware provided by the bartenders, but instead gulped from an enormously thick plastic cup – the kind they fill with soft drinks in football stadiums and sell for four or five dollars each – except her cup contained much more Jack Daniels than soft drink. Between drags from the container squeezed between quivering jealous hands, Darla

Bender glanced at her watch with exasperation, alternating darting glares between her former lover and his child-bride and the rear area of the property beyond the pool.

On the periphery of the dance area, Yvette and the smaller catering firms involved had installed round tables covered with white linens and adorned them with bowls of nuts and other more casual pickup foods. Hobby Dencil sat alone at one of those tables – drinking, drinking hard. He had tipped one of the circulating beverage servers to keep his cosmopolitan topped off. The alcohol numbed the humiliation of the embarrassing spectacle before him made worse by the house he had allowed to happen and had grown to hate. With each gulp of his never ending cosmo, he wondered why he had come to the party in the first place. However, he had to see it; he had to punish himself.

"Great wallpaper in the garden room, Hobby," his nemesis from Baton Rouge had slyly said after slipping up behind him in the food serving line. As he shoveled a generous serving of tenderloin from the mahogany banquet table, the competing architect knew full well that Rachel Pixler's color of green had persuaded Dencil to use such an unorthodox design.

"I've never seen a floor design like that," another decorator, that one from Atlanta, had said to Dencil in sarcastic reference to the library as she perused the dessert selection. Choosing a lemon square drizzled with honey, she added a wink of ridicule for the hideous busts of the Pixlers which trounced that same room beyond repair. Resurrecting the idea for his and her Pixler busts, Rachel had them secretly commissioned in France and sprung the things on Dencil a few days before the party. They stood on marble pedestals, ruling Manorwood Heights and blocking the view through the added library window.

It was now nearly midnight, about an hour before the band was to stop. The crowd had thinned considerably since Kaylee and I had unexpectedly bumped into Granddad and the gynecologist's widow. Fortunately, they had left nearly an hour previously. As expected, those still in attendance had remained congregated outside to the rear. After his sixth cosmo, Dencil neared an out-of-body experience as he sat alone at his patio table. He had survived the ordeal by imagining himself in New York or London or even Mexico, anywhere but at the Pixler Palace in Larkspur, Mississippi. In defiance, the remainder of the guests appeared overjoyed to be at the home of Cordell and Rachel Pixler; they continued dancing, drinking, flirting, and laughing as though a ritual. A few particularly happy ones had even taken a spontaneous swim in the Pixlers' pool and then had stripped down, leaving enough layers to prevent total indecent exposure.

He had devised something simple, and since detailed advance surveillance of the house had been impossible, he chose the phone system. Even though cell phone use was rampant by then, a house that size would have had landlines at least for security reasons. Why the clothes that he saw from afar were left hanging from the fence at the rear of the property, he never understood. However, finding the abandoned white caterer's uniform had been a last minute, unexpected bonus, although definitely a snug fit. Disguised as one of the food servers, the smooth execution of the plan was therefore facilitated by giving him access to almost the entire first and second floors. Yvette's ignorance of that employee substitution for Wayne Simmons was guaranteed by her attention to keeping Faith glued to the fabulous crab bisque.

Moving through the confusion of the boisterous party, which earlier in the evening was centered more inside the mansion than at the rear, he had ample opportunity for contact with the phone system. While bending to retrieve partially consumed crackers or chocolate-dipped strawberries dropped by careless guests or while picking up dirty glasses, utensils, or wadded party napkins, he slipped a DSL filter on as many units as he could reach. Employing the one-inch square plastic devices as inconspicuous connectors along a phone cord as it leaves the wall outlet was the perfect way to provide the ignition source for a tremendous fire. And since the Pixlers had a lot of surface phones to enable an intricate intercom system, there would be multiple points of origin.

He had equipped each DSL filter with an electronic match and enough C4 plastic explosive to blow a small table apart, carrying the diminutive supplies in the side pockets of the abandoned caterer's outfit. Since all wires and cords and connectors had been installed as inconspicuously as possible to please Mrs. Cordell Pixler, it was possible to hide the DSL ignition devices behind or under furniture or drapery, perfect as combustion sources when the C4 would come alive. He even stole a moment to install a few of the diminutive, but powerful, bombs upstairs when an elderly guest asked him to help her to a vacant ladies' room there.

Ringing one of the phone landlines would supply seventy watts of electrical power, an ample source to trigger the ignition of a series of small but carefully placed fires around the house. Disconnecting the phone lines while the DSL pigtails were put in place had been a concern, but a quick trip inside an electrical control room near the back stairs had accomplished that as well as providing a chance to disarm the fire alarm and security systems permanently. All of that stealth was accomplished in less than the fifteen minutes before the appointed hour.

At midnight the interior lights flickered a couple of times, then entered a psychedelic rhythm before fading into total darkness. The gamble at that moment was that no one remained upstairs, but he had already made certain of that. There were a few expected screams of surprise followed by more inebriated laughter before those remaining downstairs moved from the murky area to the still lit pool and patio. Remembering the stash of gasoline, Faith knew this was her chance to get away from the damned crab bisque, but her alarm at the pitch black surrounding forced her to search for comfort with the masses outside. Because the exterior electric outlets had been left hot, there was indeed comfort in the lively music of Pinkie and the Panthers which continued to float from the pool's center.

It was exactly 12:23 a.m. when the only remaining live landline at the Pixler Palace rang for the final time. The C4 did its job and the Palace lit up like Cinderella's Castle during a fireworks display at Walt Disney World. An added bonus to the success of the mission was an explosion near a window in the laundry room, courtesy of some gasoline-filled containers that someone had left behind.

The one person who never made it inside the Pixler residence that evening was Wayne Simmons. After trotting from the white van through the backyard to retrieve his arson supplies, he reached the tall, ivy-burdened cyclone fence at the property's rear. Fearful that he would soil his starched caterer's uniform when climbing the barrier, he stripped to his underwear and hung the outfit carefully on a post. Once over the fence, he opened the cabinet attached to the Ridley garage where he had stored the equipment. Bending down to thoroughly search the dim space, he found the Party Happy candles but not the rest of his stuff. "Where the hell is the damn brake fluid?" Simmons cursed almost loud enough to be heard back at the palace. The brake fluid was to be an essential supplement to the other fire ignition sources. It would fill the kitchen coffee maker canisters and those found in the private bedroom suites.

"What brake fluid?" a voice from around the corner interrupted.

"The brake fluid I left it in the fuckin' car trunk," he answered absent-mindedly before jerking up to realize that he was not alone.

A female police officer had rounded the corner from the garage and stared at him hungrily, as though prey. Her shiny uniform badge read *L. Sleethe* and was pinned near an embroidered patch bragging *LARKSPUR, THE FRIENDLY HOMETOWN.* Wayne had never faced a policewoman with bright red lips and false eyelashes, especially a perfumed example who walked stiffly as though her body were in a vise. Regardless of the officer's appearance, the moment was an unfortunate slice of fate for Wayne Simmons. Knowing that the Ridley residence was unoccupied, she had been careful to patrol that alley daily near dark. A charge of trespassing, vagrancy, and lewdness would help monthly ticket and arrest production for Officer Lyric Sleethe. She needed a promotion and salary raise to fund the cosmetics and off-duty clothing accumulated with the coerced assistance of Minor Leblanc.

As a result, Wayne Simmons became preoccupied with other issues, so Darla Bender never again heard from him. Per Simmons' arson-services policy, there was no reason for further contact since she had paid him in advance, in full, and had received what she had ordered during the cellular call to Memphis: the destruction of the mansion by fire. Although she had expected the evening's blaze to originate sooner during the night, Bender was satisfied because she had unquestionably gotten her money's worth. However, unbeknownst to her someone else did the work.

Likewise, Faith Behneman vicariously achieved her goal of material harm to the lawyer she saw as unjustly successful at her expense. Running clear of Pixler's burning house, she smiled as an explosion emanated from the laundry room, fueled separately by the abandoned gasoline-filled plastic containers.

The initial plan for the inferno that inadvertently pleased Bender

and Behneman had actually been my teacher's idea, concocted
during one of our late-night heart-to-heart talks at the fire station.
And as expected, Alvin Coakley did a thorough job that night
at the Pixler Palace fundraiser, a job with doubled significance.
During one of his initial visits to Larkspur, I had privately shared
the whole miserable story of the Foxworth family downfall as
Coakley absorbed every resentful sentence. He himself had never
liked lawyers, principally a fairly inexperienced specimen who
ruthlessly removed him from the training faculty at the Bureau
of Alcohol, Tobacco, and Firearms. While initially I believed Al's
objective to be avenging my family's destruction at the hands of a
conniving lawyer, I learned of his own deep desire for retaliation.
Along crushing legal lines, our paths had deeply connected. The
attorney at his ATF arbitration had been a young Ole Miss law
school graduate named Cordell Pixler who had gained admission
to the California Bar and hoped for a star-studded career on the
West Coast.

Al Coakley jumped at the chance to torch the Pixler Palace as
we shared equal pleasure in getting even with the blood-sucker.
While my part was to make the cell phone call at exactly 12:23 a.m.
when supposedly using the men's room, I thought about calling
the whole thing off when I saw happy Granddad at the party with
Madelyn Gwinn. But then I envisioned my miserable father and
mother, emotionally tortured by the death of that poor teenage
girl who died under Dad's care; they had been completely ruined
by the ruthless, seemingly vindictive lawyer. Whether my parents'
deadly plane crash had been a byproduct of all that, who was to
know? But I could not help believing that to be the case.

Occasionally the guilt over what I did to the Pixlers bothers
me, although there was something so definitive and satisfying
about what was done that night. That same sense of gratification
resurfaces each time I sit before a roaring fireplace or see a buddy

light a cigar after a pricey, satisfying meal. Regardless, the remorse over abandoning principles taught me by my parents has been simple to overcome. Volunteering my services as a physician through the Soup Kitchen in Jackson has thoroughly served that purpose. I also do a certain amount of medical work gratis in my own plastic surgery practice.

I especially like to help burn victims.

Epilogue

The investigation of the Pixler fire was never solved. Alvin Coakley, after all, was the principal fire investigator. As per our agreement, he and I never discussed what we had executed so thoroughly that night at the school fundraiser. And our pact will remain unbroken since my dear friend succumbed a few years later to cirrhosis of the liver, an aftereffect of his earlier days.

The Pixlers received a generous insurance settlement for their loss, although Cordell certainly could have done without it. In fact the monetary settlement was so equitable that many in Larkspur and vicinity blamed the good lawyer himself for the blaze. Some even believed he wore a guilty look on his face for several months; I prefer to think of it as frightened. The couple never rebuilt on the hilly site, and I think that at some point the young golddigger Rachel joined his list of divorced wives.

With the help of the admissions test review course, I finally made it to medical school a couple of years after the bonfire. For once, my MCAT was high enough, and according to the admissions committee, I had achieved a worthy level of maturity. Kaylee and I then married after I completed first-year gross anatomy, because she abhorred the permeating smell of formaldehyde.

Granddad's backyard, squirrels and all, was a fantastic place for our wedding reception where the former Madelyn Gwinn was a smooth stand-in for both my mother and Memaw. Few people wind up with a step-grandmother, but I was thankful for mine and thrilled for Senior. After redecoration and the return of love and much-needed laughter, his old house had become their happy, new home. Otherwise left unaltered, my father's teenage room came alive within that vibrant atmosphere as it received a daily dusting and vase of fresh greenery, both courtesy of Madelyn Gwinn Foxworth.

Marriage, to the contrary, still eludes Officer Lyric Sleethe although she has explored every relationship opportunity. Upon the arrest of Wayne Simmons, she handcuffed him per procedure and stuck him in the back of her squad car where I had ridden so uncomfortably before. However, Sleethe admired the way Simmons carried his boxers and wife-beater tee and gave him a choice of options: booking and certain jail time or a country road romp with a policewoman and her bright red lips. Simmons chose the latter under the condition she buy him some replacement clothes at Wal-Mart since his caterer's uniform was left on the Pixler side of the fence. Afterwards, he escaped through the exterior window of a convenience store men's room; he never again wanted to have sex in the backseat of a squad car.

While Wayne Simmons has yet to return to Lyric Sleethe and Larkspur, I have essentially never left the town. I successfully resurrected my father's booming plastic surgery practice and remain a model citizen even in the eyes of the clueless police, all except one. So like a model Larkspurian, I occasionally drive by that still-empty lot in Manorwood Heights to keep an eye on the place where the palace once stood.

Except for a few raccoons and a possum or two, nothing remains to grace that hill save for the native animals' scavenger hunt for half-eaten Krystals and cold French fries. The neighborhood security patrol scatters the stream of littering teenagers who continue to ignore the *POSTED - NO TRESPASSING* marker, the teenagers who think nothing of defaming the previously spectacular area with their paper wrappers, body wastes, and other rubbish. Likewise, broken liquor bottles and beer cans are left peeking from the stagnant water at the base of a once majestic but now abandoned pool, the same pool that supported Pinkie and her clan.

Even though the bulldozers cleared away the charred debris of the enormous fire, the flagstone steps leading from the road toward the front of the Pixler Palace survived. Sometimes I walk the dog down the street that runs in front of those remaining steps. However, it's not Dickens anymore that I walk. Poor old thing just couldn't hold on any longer, but he had lived a full life – a hero's life.

While one cannot fully replace a beloved pet, particularly one inherited in the manner in which that old Chinese pug fell to me, I did get another dog, a different type even smaller but still noisy, a Chihuahua. Her name is Mariquita; a nice fellow who speaks Spanish suggested the name. Because pet adoption had worked nicely for me in the past, and since I was not aware of any shut-ins awaiting rescue from a burning house, I adopted Mariquita from the Mississippi Animal Rescue League down in Jackson. She was only three or four months old when I got her, having been found abandoned on the side of a country road. And I think I know why: she remains impossible to house train although Mari (sometimes I call her Quita) is a really sweet animal. Maybe by this time next year, Quita will have had no sneakily planned accidents for at least two days in a row. But I'm not optimistic.

Like dear-departed Dickens, Mariquita likes to walk for recreation and unlike some Chihuahuas easily accepts a leash. With increased speed she actually seems to pull against it as we approach the Pixler property. Reaching the bottom of the flagstone steps, Quita eagerly leads me up them, similarly ignoring the *POSTED - NO TRESPASSING* sign hanging askew from an unscathed gigantic oak. Even though her legs are thin and short, my new dog relishes in ascending the monumental staircase, the one that previously beckoned the curious and the jealous to the Pixler Palace.

Step by step we climb, until we reach the top – and we're pretty good at it.

THE END

About the Author

Darden North, MD, is an obstetrician/gynecologist who lives in Jackson, Mississippi, where he practices medicine at the Jackson Healthcare for Women, PA. He and his wife Sally have two children, a college age son and daughter, as well as two dogs, a cat, and a granddog.

North's first novel, *House Call*, was published in October 2005.

REFERENCES

DeHann, John D. Kirk's *Fire Investigation, Fifth Edition.* Upper Saddle River, New Jersey: Prentice Hall, 2002

Corporate Investigative Services. *Fire Investigations & Failure Analysis Related to Fire & Explosion Accident & Crash Reconstruction* 21 June 2004. 11 Nov. 2005 <http://www.arson-codes.com/library/index.shtml>

Churchward, Daniel. "Fire Investigation: A Thirty-Year Perspective." Insurance Committee for Arson Control Keynote Speech. San Antonio, TX, Jan. 2003

Hines, Lora. "Insurance Fund Broke; Victims in Limbo." *The Clarion Ledger* 18 Nov. 2005, Sec. A2

"Airplane Icing." *The National Center for Atmospheric Research & the UCAR Office.* 5 July 2005. 11 Nov. 2005 <http://www.ucar.edu/research/society/icing.shtml>

Sharma, Sat, MD, FRCPC, FACP, FCCP, DABSM. *eMedicine – Pulmonary Embolism.* 3 June 2005. 10 Dec. 20 <http://www.emedicine.com/med/topic1958.htm>